Living with Eczema

Mom Asks, Doc Answers!

Living with Eczema

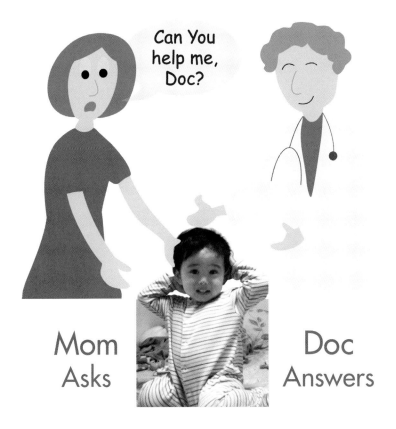

Mom
Asks

Doc
Answers

Hugo Van Bever, MD, PhD

National University of Singapore, Singapore

MarcieMom

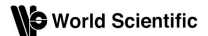 **World Scientific**

NEW JERSEY · LONDON · SINGAPORE · BEIJING · SHANGHAI · HONG KONG · TAIPEI · CHENNAI

Published by

World Scientific Publishing Co. Pte. Ltd.
5 Toh Tuck Link, Singapore 596224
USA office: 27 Warren Street, Suite 401-402, Hackensack, NJ 07601
UK office: 57 Shelton Street, Covent Garden, London WC2H 9HE

Book cover illustrated by MarcieMom (Yee, Mei Hua)
Website for this book: http://EczemaQnA.com

Library of Congress Cataloging-in-Publication Data
Van Bever, Hugo, author.
  Living with eczema : mom asks, doc answers! / Hugo Van Bever, MarcieMom.
   p. ; cm.
  Includes index.
  ISBN-13: 978-9814590716 (hardcover : alk. paper)
  ISBN-10: 9814590711 (hardcover : alk. paper)
  ISBN-13: 978-9814579513 (pbk. : alk. paper)
  ISBN-10: 9814579513 (pbk. : alk. paper)
  I. MarcieMom, author. II. Title.
  [DNLM: 1. Dermatitis, Atopic. 2. Eczema. 3. Physician-Patient Relations. WR 160]
  RL251
  616.5'1--dc23
                                        2013047885

British Library Cataloguing-in-Publication Data
A catalogue record for this book is available from the British Library.

Printed in Singapore by Mainland Press Pte Ltd.

We dedicate this book to
all children with eczema and
their families and hope that
this book will help all of them.

Foreword

In this book, Mei (also known as MarcieMom and mother of a child with atopic eczema), and Professor Hugo (a pediatric allergist with an interest in atopic eczema) come together in a most interesting way to try and dispel a lot of the ignorance and myths about eczema and its different types. Each chapter starts off with some facts and theories which then trigger a series of questions by Mei which are then answered by Professor Hugo. It is a dialogue that works well in that it gives the reader insights into both the person asking the question and the person providing the answer, and it promotes shared decision making between patients and healthcare professionals. I also like the strong emphasis on quality of life and psychological factors of eczema in this guide, which is supplemented by practical advice when the evidence on what to do is not that clear. The book covers important areas that are commonly asked about during eczema consultations such as the importance of the skin barrier, what is safe and not safe in terms of treatment, and the role of food allergies which is often overplayed. The book also usefully tackles eczema in adults which is another rather neglected area. Given that eczema is on the increase worldwide, this book is a timely and practical resource for everyone interested in atopic eczema.

Professor Hywel Williams
Director
Centre of Evidence-Based Dermatology
University of Nottingham
UK

Foreword

Eczema is a common manifestation of allergies in children. Poor or inadequate control of the disease can significantly impact on the quality of life of the child and even the family. The approach to optimal care and management requires a multidisciplinary approach. Having a good understanding of the steps involved in eczema care, and dispelling myths are vital in the management of this condition.

This book provides a light-hearted approach to the essential facts that every patient and caregiver should be familiar with. The presentation makes for easy reading and enables the reader to identify with the clearly organised issues in a systematic manner that is easily understood. The practical approach will certainly benefit patients and positively impact on the overall outlook of their conditions. Congratulations on a fantastic effort, one that I am sure the patients and their caregivers will appreciate.

Professor Daniel Goh
Head of Department of Paediatrics
National University of Singapore

Contents

Introduction

Atopic eczema or atopic dermatitis (AD) (i.e. eczema in which allergy is involved) is the most common chronic skin disease in children, affecting up to 20% worldwide, especially during the first years of life. Recent data from epidemiological studies suggest that there is still an increase in the prevalence of AD, especially in developed countries. AD is made up of different subtypes, and based on different underlying mechanisms, but all resulting in a chronic inflammation of the skin, which is the hallmark of AD. The complete underlying mechanisms of AD are still fairly unknown. AD is considered to be a complex disease in which a number of abnormalities play a role. These include: skin barrier dysfunctions, allergies, immune abnormalities, and abnormal skin colonisation with bacteria, affecting normal human microbiota.

I have been treating eczema patients for the last 30 years, and I have experienced that AD can be a very terrible disease, leading to desperation and having a huge impact on quality of life of the child and the whole family. AD affects the outside (i.e. the appearance), and is therefore, at least, an embarrassing disease. Moreover, AD induces a constant itch, resulting in extensive scratching, sleep disturbances, even learning problems for children. The psychological trauma induced by AD easily leads to social isolation.

Recently, good progress has been made in understanding underlying mechanisms, but a lot of questions still exist. The results of most recent studies in AD point to the role of the skin barrier as an initial abnormality in AD. This book aims to present the latest, comprehensive information on AD, and be a valuable resource for patients, parents and various practitioners.

Professor Hugo Van Bever

Eczema is a condition that I will not wish on any child, having gone through the experience of taking care of a child with eczema from two weeks old. When my baby was first diagnosed with eczema, many questions started rolling in, from 'Why did my child get eczema?' to 'How do I help her with the itch?' The more I tried to find out, the more questions I had. That is why I'm committed and passionate about this book, and grateful that I have the privilege of working on this book and asking Professor Hugo questions that will help with managing important aspects of life with eczema. I also thank Professor Hywel Williams and Amanda Roberts from the Nottingham Support Group for Carers of Children with Eczema for the support they have provided for this book. Many eczema sufferers and parents of children with eczema have kindly volunteered their pictures and help to spread the word of this book and I'm greatful for your participation. Lastly, thank you to MarcieDad who supported me lovingly to raise Marcie, who is an inspiration for my eczema work.

Mei, also known as MarcieMom of EczemaBlues.com

Aim of the Book

This book is built up as a conversation between a mother of a child with AD and the doctor who is treating the child. In that way, the book aims to answer different types of questions that parents (as well as patients and doctors) might have on AD. Hereby, the book will offer practical information on AD, but also cover recent research findings on AD. The ultimate aim of this book is to be a useful source of information for people suffering from AD, parents of children who suffer from AD and practitioners who treat AD. In brief, for everybody interested in AD.

PART

Learning about Eczema

CHAPTER 1

Eczema Basics

Definition

Eczema is an inflammatory skin condition, characterised by ichtyosis (dry skin), erythema (redness), excoriation (interruption of the skin), scratching lesions, lichenification (thickening of the skin), infected lesions (blisters, pus formation), and hypopigmentation or hyperpigmentation in old lesions. Eczema is now considered as a group of chronic skin diseases, of which allergic eczema or atopic dermatitis (AD) is the most common type in children (i.e. eczema in which allergy is involved).

The most Common Types of Eczema (Overlap Exists)

1. Atopic dermatitis
2. Constitutional eczema
3. Contact dermatitis
4. Seborrhoeic eczema

Other Types of Eczema

Eczema is a syndrome (i.e. a group of chronic skin diseases with similar clinical features) of which allergic eczema or atopic dermatitis (AD) is the most common type. AD is chronic eczema in which allergy is involved. Other types of eczema include *constitutional eczema* (eczema without signs of allergy), *seborrhoeic eczema* and *contact eczema*. A distinction between atopic eczema and constitutional (or intrinsic) eczema, based on the presence or absence of an underlying allergy, can be temporal, as eczema can develop prior to allergy in children. In infants from allergic families without evidence of an underlying allergy (but who are expected to become allergic after prolonged exposure to allergens), the term pre-allergic eczema might be used, although not generally accepted. Other types of eczema have been described, merely based on clinical presentation, less on underlying mechanisms. Recently, it was proposed to revise the nomenclature on eczema and to replace the term AD by atopic eczema/dermatitis syndrome (AEDS).

Seborrhoeic Eczema

This type of eczema appears in infants, usually between two weeks to two months of life as red, scaly rashes on the trunk (back) and scalp. The lesions are red and crusty, and there can be a yellowish scaly crust on the scalp (known as cradle cap). Sometimes, distinguishing from early AD is difficult, even impossible. However, this type of eczema has a better prognosis, as most infants will recover very quickly, as a consequence of a local treatment. Some children with seborrhoeic eczema will develop atopic dermatitis later, and a link between the two types of eczema is suspected. The underlying mechanisms of seborrhoeic eczema are fairly unknown. For some researchers, this type of eczema has the same underlying mechanisms as AD, and is also closely linked with an underlying atopic constitution. The main treatments for infants are emollient creams, but mild corticosteroid creams may be needed. Cradle cap, which is a

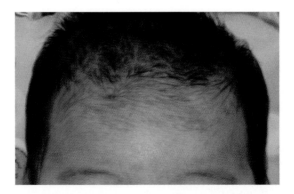

Fig. 1.1 Cradle cap as a mild manifestation of seborrhoeic dermatitis, which is associated with atopic dermatitis.

manifestation of seborrhoeic eczema, can be loosened with a mixture of salicylic acid in a moisturiser, which is then washed out with baby shampoo. Oils such as olive oil are also long-standing remedies for de-scaling cradle cap. Seborrhoeic eczema can also occur in older children and during adulthood, although it is not sure whether the underlying mechanisms are similar as those in infants.

Contact Eczema or Contact Dermatitis

Contact eczema is a localised rash or irritation of the skin caused by an inflammation of the skin, as a result of direct contact of the skin with a foreign substance. IgE (i.e. the immunoglobulin involved in allergy) is not involved in contact dermatitis, as this is a delayed type of immune response (type IV immune response) in which lymphocytes (called T cells) are activated.

Contact dermatitis in children is increasing. This seems to be independent from the increase of allergic diseases. However, an indirect reason for its increase could be that contact dermatitis is more common in children with atopic dermatitis, due to the use of topical products in children with AD who are sensitive to certain ingredients in the moisturisers and lotions.

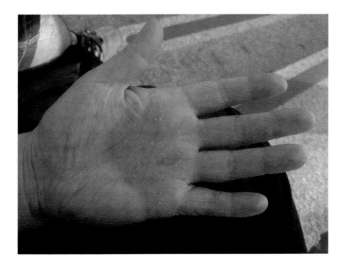

Fig. 1.2   Contact dermatitis on hand of adult due to contact with chemicals on the job.

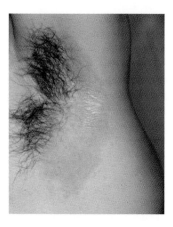

Fig. 1.3   Contact dermatitis due to deodorant spray.

Other possible reasons for the increase are: (1) an increased awareness for the problem, and (2) the fact that we use more skin products (cosmetic products) than in the past, including an increased use of soaps and cleaning products, which might affect the integrity of the skin barrier.

Sensitisation to contact allergens may already begin at an early age, but data on the prevalence of contact eczema in young children in the general population are unavailable. However, it is generally accepted that the prevalence of contact eczema is lower than that of atopic dermatitis. In contrast, the contact sensitisation rate increases with age, as environmental exposures accumulate.

Substances that cause contact dermatitis in many people include "poisonous" plants such as poison ivy, metals (nickel, such as in jewellery or piercings), cleaning solutions, detergents, cosmetics, perfumes, leather (shoes) and industrial chemicals. Avoidance of the substance is the most effective treatment. Local application of corticosteroids reduces the inflammation.

The golden standard in diagnosing contact eczema is the *skin patch test*. However, limited experience in young children (i.e. normal values) is still a problem. From the available literature it is accepted that the most common contact in children are: metals (nickel), fragrances, preservatives, neomycin, rubber chemicals and p-tert-butyl-phenol-formaldehyde resin.

Factors inducing contact dermatitis in children

1. Filaggrin (FLG) deficiency (loss-of-function) is a risk for both atopic dermatitis and contact dermatitis, the latter occurring more frequently by allowing easier contact of haptens with the epidermal immune system (including the antigen-presenting cells). Reports on nickel-induced contact eczema have been published. However, it is accepted that FLG has a more important role in atopic dermatitis.

2. Atopic dermatitis is a risk for contact dermatitis, but results of studies on the association between both types of eczema are still controversial. However, most researchers agree that the role of contact allergy in AD is frequently underestimated. Therefore, preventive measures in children with AD should be introduced. These include: avoidance of nickel-containing objects, perfumed cosmetics, and topical medication containing lanolin and neomycin. Antiseptics, such as chlorhexidine, corticosteroids and emollients are other potential causes of contact dermatitis but remain conventional treatments for AD, due to efficacy.

Epidemiology, Symptoms and Prognosis of AD

Epidemiology

The prevalence of AD is the highest in infancy, and the natural course of most patients with AD is remission during childhood. In Singapore, AD affects about 20% of young children below the age of two years. Worldwide, there has been an increase in prevalence of AD during the last 30 years worldwide (as shown in the ISAAC studies), which is in parallel with the increase of prevalence of atopy. In older children the prevalence of AD is lower, usually between 10–15% of children.

Symptoms

AD has no specific skin signs and is a result of chronic skin inflammation. The lesions are non-typical and are made up of dry skin, red spots, crusts (pointing to interruption of the skin), scratching lesions, thickening of the skin, infected lesions (blisters, pus formation), and hypopigmentation or hyperpigmentation in old lesions. The diagnosis of AD is usually based on clinical assessment and on established criteria, such as the criteria of Hanifin and Rajka.

Except for dry skin, children do not have symptoms from birth. The first symptoms of AD usually appear before the age of three months. The exact triggers of the first lesions of AD are unknown, but recently the role of skin microbiota has been highlighted (i.e. due to congenital skin barrier defects, AD infants are not able to build up a normal diverse skin flora, causing inflammation). Usually, allergic reactions are not present at that early age. In 80% of children with AD, the lesions appear before the age of one year and in 90% before the age of five years. The most invariable symptom is ITCH (= **pruritus**), which can be very intense. The distribution profile of the disease varies with age and is characterised by the predominance of certain skin lesions.

Infants

The areas most commonly affected are the face, scalp, neck, arms and legs (especially the front of the knees and the back of the elbows), and trunk.

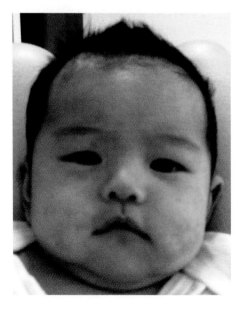

Fig. 1.4 Baby with eczema on the face at four months old.

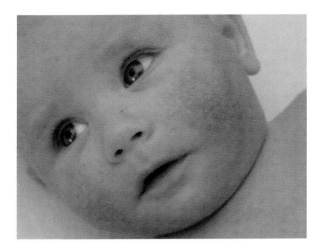

Fig. 1.5 Eczema on infant's cheeks.

The rash usually does not appear in the diaper area. The rash presents most commonly as dry, red, scaling areas on the baby's cheeks. The rash is often crusted or oozes fluid, and rubbing and scratching can lead to frequent infections.

Older children (age 2 to 11 years)

The symptoms may appear for the first time or may be a continuation of the infant phase. The rash occurs primarily on the back of the legs and arms, on the neck, and in areas that bend, such as the back of the knees and the inside of the elbows. Wrists and ankles are also commonly involved. The rash is usually dry. But it may go through stages from an acute oozing rash to a red, dry subacute rash to a chronic rash that causes the skin to thicken (lichenification). Lichenification often occurs after the rash goes away. Rubbing and scratching can lead to infections.

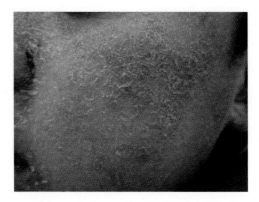

Fig. 1.6 An older child with dry rash.

Adolescents and adults

AD often improves as children get older. The areas affected by atopic dermatitis are usually small and commonly include places that bend, such as the neck, the back of the knees, and the inside of the elbows. Rashes can also affect the face, wrists, and forearms. Rashes are rare in the groin area. Usually the skin remains very dry, with hyperlinearity of hands and feet, and with pronounced lichenification.

The diagnosis of AD is generally not difficult, but in some cases the symptoms are poorly defined. In this event the diagnostic criteria of

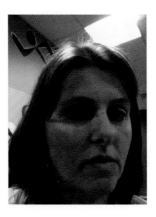

Fig. 1.7 An adult with facial eczema.

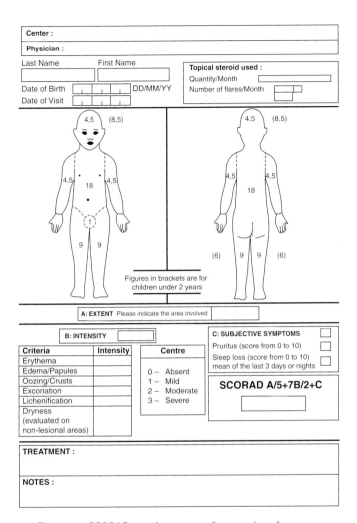

Fig. 1.8 SCORAD, scoring system for severity of eczema.

Hanifin and Lobitz (or Rajka) are useful. These criteria are well known and used by clinicians all over the world. The severity of AD can be assessed by usage of the scoring system SCORAD (Fig. 1.8), which is of importance in follow-up of the disease or in standardisation of criteria of severity as needed in clinical trials. The clinical course is characterised by variability and unpredictability. The asymptomatic intervals usually become extended as the child ages.

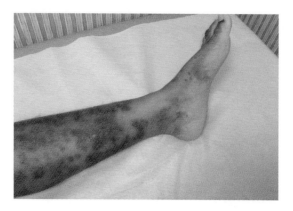

Fig. 1.9 Hyperpigmented lesions as a consequence of eczema.

Prognosis

In most children the prognosis of AD is favourable, as most of them will grow out of their skin problems. However, about one in three children with AD will develop respiratory allergy (asthma or rhinitis) later in life (50% in children with severe AD). Usually, AD gets better when the child gets older, but many children with severe AD have persistent lesions for many years, and in some the lesions will persist during adulthood. In most cases, there is a decrease in flare-ups of acute exacerbations, and the symptom-free intervals get longer, although the dryness of the skin remains. It has been shown in follow-up studies that 60% of children with severe AD will still have symptoms at the age of 20. In more than 90% of children with mild to moderate AD, symptoms disappear before the age of 20. Most adults who suffered from AD during childhood will still have a persistence of dry and itchy skin. Moreover, under-treated AD can lead to the persistence of severe rest lesions (scaring of the skin). The rest lesions of AD are usually hyper-pigmented lesions for which there is no treatment.

Mom Asks, Doc Answers!

MarcieMom: *Professor Hugo, if a child has dry skin and feels itchy but there is no sign of rashes, would that be considered eczema?*

Professor Hugo: Yes, as eczema affects the whole skin and can be unnoticed, let's say: microscopically or subclinical. What you see is the top of the iceberg, but under the surface the lesions can be present. However, we advise that only the visible lesions are treated. If there is only dry skin, we advise to moisturise.

MarcieMom: *Does the presence of dry skin indicate that the child will have eczema?*

Professor Hugo: Not necessarily. A dry skin suggests an abnormal skin barrier, and is a risk for eczema. However, not all children with dry skin will develop eczema. Other factors, some still unknown, are necessary to develop eczema.

MarcieMom: *What does inflamed skin looks like? Why does the skin get inflamed, and is it possible to have inflammation in the lower layers of skin and not be visible to the human eye?*

Professor Hugo: In AD, inflammation can be everywhere, but, according to age, more in certain areas (see text). The main symptom of inflammation of the skin is redness, causing itch. It is the rash that itches, according to some. The cause of the inflammation is abnormal underlying immune responses, which can be caused by allergic reactions in some children.

MarcieMom: *As a moderator of an eczema forum, I have come across a mother asking if her child has eczema when there is rash but the child is not scratching, i.e. not feeling itchy at all! Is this possible?*

Professor Hugo: Most eczema is itchy, but exceptions do occur. If the skin is red, it means inflammation is present, and treatment is needed.

MarcieMom: *You mentioned about constitutional eczema (i.e. eczema without signs of allergy). Is it possible that there is an allergic reaction but cannot be captured by allergy testing due to the limitations of the tests?*

Professor Hugo: This is possible but very unlikely, as our current allergy testing is sensitive enough to pick up allergies. However, at the onset of an allergy it can be that it is not picked up. If the eczema persists or gets worse, I advise to repeat the tests after six months to a year. This is on condition that the correct allergy test (using the appropriate allergens) is used.

MarcieMom: *How does one differentiate seborrhoeic eczema from dandruff?*

Professor Hugo: Dandruff usually causes no inflammation of the skin, meaning no redness. However, mild seborrhoeic eczema (cradle cap) can sometimes present as dandruff. The treatment is similar.

MarcieMom: *Seborrhoeic eczema on the scalp is often associated with allergic reaction to a yeast, called Malassezia furfur, a form of yeast that is commonly found on areas with more sebaceous glands as it requires fats to grow. Are individuals with oily skin or scalps then more likely to have seborrhoeic eczema, i.e. the more oil, the more yeast, the higher the likelihood to be sensitised to it?*

Professor Hugo: This is mainly an adult problem. In children yeasts are usually not involved in eczema, although exceptions exist. Special culturing is necessary to show the presence of yeasts in the skin. Having an oily skin can be a risk for seborrhoeic eczema in adults, but not a necessity. This is extremely uncommon in children.

MarcieMom: *My child had cradle cap that developed at about one month old and got very crusty. I followed the pediatrician's instruction to rub the crust with olive oil and then de-scaled the crust. Once, I left the olive oil on the scalp as my baby fell asleep half-way through the "soaking" and she woke up with a terribly red and itchy scalp. Is it possible that the olive oil is an irritant to her scalp?*

Professor Hugo: Olive oil is safe, and there is no data to support the hypothesis that fragrances or preservatives can induce atopic eczema in children. Spontaneous reports of contact dermatitis have been published, but this is uncommon.

MarcieMom: *From an eczema forum, I have come across an individual with contact eczema that persists despite the avoidance of the substance. Could the initial inflammation of skin lead to a weakened skin barrier at the contact point, which then results in the individual being vulnerable to other irritants?*

Professor Hugo: Yes, this is possible, as inflammation on itself can also induce skin barrier dysfunctions. However, sometimes contact dermatitis needs time to settle, even after removal of the substance.

MarcieMom: *You also mentioned that eczema does not commonly occur at the diaper area for infants. Why is this so? How would a parent differentiate diaper rash from eczema rash? Is urine a possible irritant that can trigger contact dermatitis?*

Professor Hugo: We don't know why eczema doesn't appear in the diaper area. Diaper rash is usually a skin irritation with inflammation, caused by urine or stools. Sometimes parents think it is eczema, but the cause is totally different.

MarcieMom: *Many parents are very worried about permanent pigmentation on patches of skin that the child constantly scratches. Some feel that the likelihood of a permanent discolouration is linked to the application of steroid cream. Can you explain what causes the discolouration?*

Professor Hugo: No, there are no scientific studies showing that local corticosteroids cause discolouration of the skin. It is the eczema lesions themselves, especially when infected, that cause hypo- and hyper-pigmentation.

MarcieMom: *Are there any factors that will predict if the child can grow out of eczema?*

Professor Hugo: The more severe the eczema, the higher the risk that it will persist. Also if the child is highly allergic (especially to house dust mites) the risk of persistence is higher. There are, however, no prognostic markers of eczema. The main message is: treat all eczema. If not, complications may occur, such as scarring and skin infections.

CHAPTER 2

Normal Skin versus Eczema Skin

Introduction

The skin is considered the largest organ of the human body and the largest contact area with the environment. The skin is a barrier with multiple functions, such as protecting, adapting, and keeping our metabolism in optimal condition, through various barrier functions, including local immune responses. In children with AD the skin is abnormal, defined as an abnormal skin barrier. The skin is made up of not only cells but also bacteria, called microbiota. It is important to note that normal skin needs bacteria to create a perfect eco-system. In children with eczema the eco-system is altered, resulting in inflammation, followed by abnormal skin colonisation, and eventually skin infections.

The Structure of Normal Skin in Children and Adults

From top to bottom, the skin consists of three layers: the epidermis, the dermis and the subcutis (also called hypodermis). The three layers differ in structure and function.

Epidermis

The epidermis is the uppermost or epithelial layer of the skin. It acts as a physical barrier, preventing loss of water from the body and entry of substances and organisms into the body. Its thickness varies according to the body site. The epidermis consists of stratified squamous epithelium. That means it consists of layers of flattened cells. In contrast to mucous membranes, skin, hair and nails are keratinised, meaning they have a dead and hardened impermeable surface made of a protein called *keratin*. The epidermis has three main types of cell:

- *Keratinocytes* (skin cells)
- *Melanocytes* (pigment-producing cells)
- *Langerhans cells* (immune cells, which present antigens to the immune system)

Keratinocytes

The keratinocytes become more mature or differentiated and accumulate keratin as they move outwards. They eventually fall or rub off. The keratinocytes form four distinct layers.

The four layers are (from the most superficial to the deepest):

1. Stratum corneum (horny layer): Consists of hard cells without nucleus.
2. Stratum granulosum (granular layer): The cells contain granules. A waxy material (i.e. skin barrier proteins) is secreted into the intercellular spaces.
3. Stratum spinosum (spiny or prickle cell layer): Intercellular bridges called desmosomes link the cells together. The cells become increasingly flattened as they move upward.
4. Stratum basale (basal layer): Consists of columnar (tall) regenerative cells. As the basal cell divides, a daughter cell migrates upwards to replenish the layer above.

Immediately below the epidermis is *the basement membrane*, which is a specialised structure that lies between the epidermis and dermis. It includes various protein structures linking the basal layer of keratinocytes to the basement membrane (hemi-desmosomes) and the basement membrane to the underlying dermis (anchoring fibrils). The basement membrane has an important role in making sure the epidermis sticks tightly to the underlying dermis. The epidermis gives rise to a number of adnexal structures. Hair and nails are both examples, i.e. they are specialised structures formed by direct extension of the epidermis. The hair follicles are associated with sebaceous (oil) glands and smooth muscle. This muscle is responsible for goose bumps appearing on the skin in response to cold or emotions. The epidermis also gives rise to sweat glands, a tangle of tubules deep within the dermis that secrete a watery salt solution into a duct that ends on the skin surface. Larger sweat glands are found in the armpits and groin.

Melanocytes

Melanocytes are found in the basal layer of the epidermis. These cells produce pigment called melanin, which is responsible for different skin colours. Melanin is packaged into small parcels (or melanosomes), which are then transferred to keratinocytes. Inflammation of the skin, as in eczema, is able to destroy the melanocytes.

Langerhans cells

Langerhans cells are immune cells found in the epidermis, and are responsible for helping the body learn and later recognise allergens. The Langerhans cells break the allergen into smaller pieces then migrate from the epidermis into the dermis. They find their way to lymphatic and blood vessels before eventually reaching the lymph nodes. Here they present the allergen to immune cells, called lymphocytes. Once the allergen is successfully "presented," the lymphocytes initiate a sequence of events to (1) initiate an immune reaction to destroy the material, and (2) stimulate proliferation of more lymphocytes that recognise and remember the allergen in the future. In eczema, abnormal immune reactions, inducing inflammation, occur.

Dermis

The dermis is the fibrous connective tissue or supportive layer of the skin. The major fibres are:

- Collagen fibres: This type of fibre predominates in the dermis. Collagen fibres have enormous tensile strength and provide the skin with strength and toughness. Collagen bundles are small in the upper or papillary dermis, and form thicker bundles in the deeper or reticular dermis.
- Elastin: This type of fibre provides the properties of elasticity and pliability to the skin.

The collagen and elastin fibres are bound together by ground substance, a mucopolysaccharide gel in which the nutrients and wastes can diffuse to and from other tissue components. The dermis also contains nerves, blood vessels, epidermal adnexal structures, and cells.

The normal cells in the dermis include:

- **Mast cells.** These contain granules packed with histamine and other chemicals, released when the cell is disturbed. These cells are activated during acute allergic reactions.
- **Vascular smooth muscle cells.** These allow blood vessels to contract and dilate, and are required to control body temperature.
- **Specialised muscle cells.** For example, myo-epithelial cells are found around sweat glands and contract to expel sweat.
- **Fibroblasts.** These are cells that produce and deposit collagen and other elements of the dermis as required for growth or to repair wounds. A resting fibroblast has very little cytoplasm compared with an active cell and appears to have a "naked" nucleus.
- **Immune cells.** There are many types of immune cells, involved in local immune responses. The role of tissue macrophages (histiocytes) is to remove and digest foreign or degraded material (this is known as phagocytosis). There are also small numbers of lymphocytes in the normal dermis.

Transient inflammatory cells or leukocytes are white cells that leave the blood vessels to heal wounds, destroy infections or cause disease, including eczema. They include:

- **Neutrophils** (polymorphs). These have segmented nuclei. They are the first white blood cells to enter tissue during acute inflammation.
- **T and B Lymphocytes**. These are small inflammatory cells with many subtypes. They arrive later but persist for longer in inflammatory skin conditions, such as eczema. They are important in the regulation of immune response. Plasma cells are specialised lymphocytes that produce different types of antibodies.
- **Eosinophils**. These have bilobed nuclei and pink cytoplasm. Eosinophils are involved in allergic reactions of the skin.
- **Monocytes**. These form macrophages.

The skin cells communicate by releasing large numbers of molecules, such as biologically active cytokines and chemotactic factors (factors that attract other cells) that regulate their function and movement.

Subcutis

The subcutis is the fat layer immediately below the dermis and epidermis. It is also called subcutaneous tissue, hypodermis or panniculus. The subcutis mainly consists of fat cells (adipocytes), nerves and blood vessels. Fat cells are organised into lobules, which are separated by structures called septae. The septae contain nerves, larger blood vessels, fibrous tissue and fibroblasts. Fibrous septae may form dimples in the skin (so-called *cellulite*).

Functions of the Skin

The skin is an organ of *protection*. The primary function of the skin is to act as a barrier. Briefly, the skin provides protection from mechanical impacts and pressure, variations in temperature, invasion by micro-organisms, radiation and chemicals. The skin is also an organ of *regulation*. The skin regulates several aspects of physiology, including: body temperature via sweat and hair, and changes in peripheral blood circulation and fluid balance via sweat. It also acts as a reservoir for the synthesis of vitamin D. The skin is an organ of *sensation*. The skin contains an extensive network of nerve cells that detect and relay changes in the environment. There are separate receptors for heat, cold, touch, and pain. Damage to these nerve cells is known as neuropathy, which results in a loss of sensation in the affected areas. Patients with neuropathy may not feel pain when they suffer injury, increasing the risk of severe wounding or the worsening of an existing wound.

Taken together, the important functions are mentioned below:

The seven important functions of the skin
1. Protection of the body
2. Sensation (transmitting information of the environment to the brain)
3. Temperature regulation
4. Immunity (role of local immune responses)
5. Enables movement and growth without injury
6. Excretion (of useless substances)
7. Endocrine function (vitamin D)

In the context of eczema, the skin has mainly a skin barrier function, which is altered in patients with eczema. This has been shown in many studies, and a lot of research on the subject is intensively ongoing. However, most of the studies were performed in adults, and it is still difficult to distinguish causal abnormalities (which are responsible for the onset of eczema) from consequential abnormalities (which are the consequence of eczema). More studies are needed in which the primary abnormalities of eczema are assessed.

For the moment, four types of skin barrier functions have been identified in a healthy skin, involving different elements of the skin (see Fig. 2.1):

1. *The physical barrier*: Made up of both the stratum corneum with its brick-and-mortar structure and the tight junctions, which are directly below the stratum corneum in the stratum granulosum.

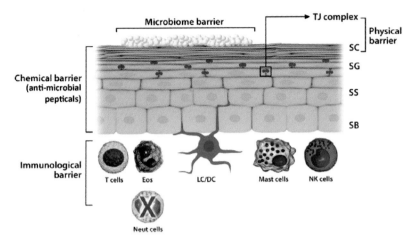

Fig. 2.1 Illustration of skin barrier layers.

Legend:
SB - Stratum basale
SC - Stratum corneum
SG - Stratum granulosum
SS - Stratum spinosum
T cells - T lymphocytes
Eos - Eosinophils
LC/DC - Langerhans cells/dendritic cells
NK - Natural killer cells
Neut - Neutrophils

2. *The chemical barrier*: Consists of a broad range of anti-microbial peptides that regulate the microbial features of the skin (commensal flora — skin microbiota).

3. *The microbioma barrier*: Consists of many bacterial, fungal, and viral phyla and subphyla. These micro-organisms play a key role in the initiation or prevention of both skin inflammation and immune responses. They protect the host from pathogens such as *Staphylococcus aureus*, which is one of the important commensals in eczema, maintaining the lesions.

4. *The immunological barrier*: Local immune responses against foreign substances, including allergens. The local immune barrier consists of two arms: an immediate, but non-specific arm (i.e. innate immunity) and a highly specific and long-lasting arm (i.e. adaptive immunity).

In subjects suffering from eczema, abnormalities in the four types of skin barrier functions have been identified. However, it is still not clear what is primary (causal) and what is secondary (consequence). Briefly, the following abnormalities of the skin barrier have been found in eczema:

1. Impaired skin barrier protein production (for the moment, the best studied protein is filaggrin).
2. Reduced expression of anti-microbial peptides.
3. Presence of allergic inflammation (accumulation of T-helper2 cells, which are the lymphocytes that orchestrate allergic reactions).
4. Defect in innate receptor functions.
5. Abnormal microbiota, especially restricted diversity of microbiota, which is considered a pro-inflammatory status and a trigger of eczema.

These are just the most important abnormalities that have been described in patients with eczema. For many years, eczema was considered primarily an immunologic disease, but more recently, epithelial barrier dysfunction has emerged as another key feature. It now becomes more and more clear that a leaky epithelial barrier might be the primary abnormality in AD, promoting allergen sensitisation and susceptibility to microbial colonisation, especially with *Staphylococcus aureus*, and even infection.

The Normal Skin at Birth

An intact healthy skin from birth is important as the first line of defense against environmental substances, including various pathogens and allergens. Although infants are born with a competent skin barrier, their skin is still developing through the first year of life, and is, therefore, different from adult skin.

The differences between infant and adult skin can be divided into structural differences, compositional differences and functional differences. The skin of newborns is drier and has a higher pH compared to that of adults, although both features are rapidly changing during the first months of life. In addition to structural and functional changes, the composition of commensal bacteria residing on the skin surface evolves during the first year of life. It is important to note that AD is not present at birth, but usually starts during the first weeks or months of life, especially in children who were born with a dry skin. The causes of the onset of AD are still unknown.

The Role of Skin Microbiota in Health and in Eczema

The human body is composed of different ecosystems, in which human cells and bacteria live in perfect harmony. The two largest eco-systems are the gastrointestinal tract and the skin.

The skin contains a large number of bacteria, living peacefully and helping to maintain the different skin functions. Recently, a lot of research has been published on the exact role of these bacteria in health and in different diseases. The skin flora, more properly referred to as the **skin microbioma** or **skin microbiota**, are the micro-organisms (bacteria, fungi, yeasts) that reside on the skin. It has been estimated that about 1000 species of bacteria are present upon human skin from more than 19 different groups or phyla. The total number of bacteria on an average human has been estimated at 10^{12} or (1,000,000,000,000). Most are found in the superficial layers of the epidermis and the upper parts of hair follicles.

Skin flora is non-pathogenic, and consists of commensals (are not harmful to their host) and mutualistic micro-organisms (offer a benefit). The benefits bacteria can offer include preventing transient pathogenic organisms from colonising the skin surface, either by competing for nutrients, secreting chemicals against them, or stimulating the skin's immune system. The latter seems to be very important in allergy and eczema. *The Hygiene Hypothesis* (Strachan, 1987) claims that the increase of allergy during the last 30 years is, at least partially, due to a decreased bacterial load (i.e. we are too clean and are destroying our favourable bacteria). However, under specific circumstances, resident microbes can cause skin diseases and enter the blood system, creating life-threatening diseases particularly in immunosuppressed people.

Recently, the role of microbiota in eczema is a subject of intensive research. More arguments are being gathered, showing that microbiota are involved in the onset of eczema and in the persistence of it. A decreased diversity of skin microbiota has been reported in children with eczema. One of the hypotheses on the causes of eczema is that infants are unable to build up normal skin microbioma, as a consequence of congenital skin barrier dysfunctions, resulting in skin inflammation. However, more studies are needed to prove this hypothesis.

Intestinal flora, also called gut flora, is the largest flora of the human body. It is an assortment of micro-organisms inhabiting the length and width of the gastrointestinal tract. The composition of this microbial community is host specific, evolving throughout an individual's lifetime and susceptible to both exogenous and endogenous modifications. Differences between children and adults have been found. Recent renewed interest in the structure and function of gut flora has illuminated its central position in health and disease. The microbiota are intimately involved in numerous aspects of normal host physiology, from nutritional status, to immune responses, to behaviour and stress response. Additionally, they can be a central or a contributing cause of many diseases, affecting both near and far organ systems. The mechanisms through which microbiota exert their beneficial or detrimental influences remain largely undefined, but include elaboration of signaling molecules and recognition of bacterial epitopes by both intestinal epithelial and local immune cells. The advances in modeling and analysis of gut microbiota will improve our knowledge of their role in health and disease, allowing customisation of existing and future therapeutic and prophylactic interventions.

Abnormalities in gut flora have been reported in children with allergies and eczema. In Singapore, we found obvious differences in gut flora between preschoolers with eczema and healthy ones. The exact mechanism on how gut microbiota influence the development of eczema are unknown, but are linked to an impact on the immune system and on skin immune responses. Moreover, it is possible that gut microbiota have an influence on skin microbiota, thereby directly inducing eczema.

The Skin in Children with Eczema

A number of alterations in skin barrier properties were described in patients with eczema. These include:

- Increased transepidermal water loss (TEWL)
- Changes in skin surface pH
- Increased skin permeability
- Altered bacterial colonisation, mainly increase in *Staphylococcus aureus* colonisation
- Compromised skin barrier integrity

The skin-barrier-function abnormalities reside mainly in the stratum corneum, being the top layer of the epidermis, and have until recently been ignored as an important factor in eczema. However, it is now clear that abnormalities of the four types of skin barrier functions exist (see above text).

TEWL measurement is performed by a non-invasive method that can be used to monitor changes in barrier function. A high TEWL is suggestive of incomplete skin barrier function. In patients with AD, TEWL was found to be increased in both dry non-eczematous skin and clinically normal skin.

Moreover, the anti-microbial barrier is compromised in AD due to an impaired expression of anti-microbial proteins (AMPs) that play a key role in the innate immune defence system of the skin. AMPs are produced by keratinocytes and the secretion of some of these peptides is constitutive, whereas the secretion of others is triggered by inflammation. Several studies showed a deficiency in the secretion of AMPs in subjects with AD. The reduced secretion of AMPs together with the observed higher pH in the skin of AD patients most likely play a role in bacterial colonisation, including colonisation with *Staphylococcus aureus*, although other abnormalities could be involved. Approximately 90% of AD patients are colonised with *S aureus* that can trigger multiple inflammatory cascades. Toxins produced by *S aureus* can act as superantigens and thereby activate inflammatory cells, such as T lymphocytes, contributing to Th2-mediated inflammatory reactions.

Different proteins of the epidermis playing an important role in the barrier function are impaired in the skin of patients with AD. Filaggrin (FLG) has been the most studied and its gene has the highest association with AD, subsequent allergic sensitisation, and allergic disorders. Next to FLG, abnormalities in other proteins expressed in the uppermost part of the epidermis have been identified to be associated with AD. These include impaired expression in tight junction proteins, such as claudins, and scaffolding proteins such as loricrin and involucrin. Importantly, the expression of these proteins can be influenced by ongoing inflammatory processes in the skin, and therefore, could be a cause or consequence of AD.

Allergens, such as house dust mites, cockroaches and *Staphylococcus aureus*, can also destroy the skin barrier.

Whether these skin barrier abnormalities are primary in the pathophysiology of AD or whether they are merely a reflection of downstream consequences of intrinsic inflammation (a consequence of eczema) remains to be fully elucidated.

Other Mechanisms Involved and a Hypothetical Model of Eczema

The development of AD is influenced by multiple factors. Genetic as well as early life environmental factors, including allergen environmental exposures, infections, autoimmunity and alcohol intake during pregnancy have been shown to be involved in eczema.

The study of epigenetic mechanisms, which means the regulation of gene expression, provides new insights on how the environment is implicated in the development of genetically determined immune-mediated diseases, including allergy, and how environmental changes drive the epidemics of allergic diseases. Although there is clear evidence that immune development is under epigenetic regulation and that alterations in epigenetic programming in allergy-prone infants are involved, little is known about epigenetic mechanisms in AD. A recent study from Liang *et al.* demonstrated a role of epigenetic changes in the pathogenesis of AD. Their results indicated demethylation of specific regulatory elements within a gene (the FCER1G gene) leading to over-expression of the high affinity IgE receptor (Fc·RI) on monocytes from patients with AD. However, further research will be required to determine the cause leading to the epigenetic changes and its potential role in the onset of AD.

Conclusion: A Hypothetical Model of Onset of AD in Early Infancy

Although progress has been made in the pathophysiology of AD, it remains a complex disorder with a complex interplay between skin barrier, immune system, skin microbioma and epigenetics (Fig. 2.2). Environmental factor-

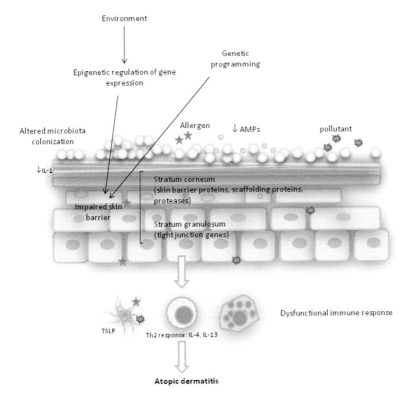

Fig. 2.2 Complex interplay between impaired skin barrier, altered skin microbiome and dysfunctional immune response in pathophysiology of AD.

induced changes in gene expression may be key in the etiology of AD. It remains to be elucidated whether epigenetic changes are causative in skin barrier impairments, leading to altered skin microbial colonisation and immune alterations or whether immune alterations are the consequence of epigenetic changes causing skin barrier dysfunction, causing increased allergen and pathogen penetration leading to AD. New insights into mechanisms underlying the onset of AD are pivotal to develop early intervention strategies to prevent the development of AD.

The onset of AD may start with an impaired skin barrier, either genetically programmed or due to specific environmental factors that via epigenetic mechanisms impair the skin barrier. The alterations in the skin barrier, physically and/or chemically, may lead to altered skin colonisation and impaired skin immune defense (e.g. reduced expression of interleukin-1 (IL-1).

Moreover, disruption of the skin barrier may enable the uptake of allergens, irritants and microbes by dendritic cells, thereby triggering inflammatory immune responses involving immune components like TSLP (thymic stromal lymphopoetin; a hormone secreted by the thymus that induces proliferation of lymphocytes, and inflammation). The inflammatory immune reaction subsequently can further impair the skin barrier functionality by decreasing the expression of skin barrier proteins like FLG, contributing to the onset of AD.

Mom Asks, Doc Answers!

MarcieMom: *Professor Hugo, for a child who is born with dry skin, should the parents immediately moisturise before the onset of eczema? Is there any study that shows a protective effect or at least a reduction in severity or delay in the onset of eczema?*

Professor Hugo: Let's say that the studies are underway. But we now accept that allergic sensitisation can occur through the skin (transdermal). Therefore, it makes sense to put an extra barrier on the skin (i.e. moisturising) to prevent transdermal sensitisation. For the moment, results of studies are not available. However, I am expecting positive results.

MarcieMom: *How does an emollient penetrate the baby's skin? For instance, do lotions penetrate deeper than creams or ointments?*

Professor Hugo: In babies, there are no studies on penetration of creams or emollients, and I am not sure whether we can use adult data in this. Even in adults there are few good comparative studies between the penetration features of creams, emollients and lotions. However, it is accepted that local treatment (on the skin) mainly affects the upper layers of the epidermis, let's say, the stratum corneum and the stratum granulosum. The main difference is the duration of contact, which is longer for ointments, resulting in a better and more sustained effect. However, most children feel more comfortable with lotions and creams than with ointments.

MarcieMom: *Which layer of skin do steroidal creams act on?*

Professor Hugo: Corticosteroids mainly act on inflammation affecting the epidermis. It is accepted that corticosteroids affect all inflammation in the epidermis, even in the dermis and hypodermis.

MarcieMom: *It is mentioned in the text that inflammation of the skin, as in eczema, is able to destroy the melanocytes. How deep in the skin layers* *does inflammation affect? Is the skin more likely to change colour the longer a person has eczema?*

Professor Hugo: In eczema, inflammation affects the epidermis and also the dermis. Corticosteroids have a global effect on all inflammation in eczema, even in the dermis. However, in severe inflammation, local corticosteroids (creams) might be insufficient. In these cases, we prescribe systemic corticosteroids (oral or even injected). Short courses are advised, as prolonged administration of systemic corticosteroids may results in side effects. The longer a person has persisted eczema, the higher the risk that the patches become infected, causing more discolouration.

MarcieMom: *It is mentioned in the text that there are collagen fibres in the dermis area. There are a lot of products marketed as reinforcing collagen. Is there any study supporting either the ingestion or the application of such products on strengthening the collagen fibres in the skin?*

Professor Hugo: No studies are available in children with eczema. However, collagen fibres seem to be unaffected in children with eczema. Collagen is mainly administered or applied against aging, but the results of the studies are rather disappointing.

MarcieMom: *For non-steroidal, topical calcineurin inhibitor creams such as tacrolimus and pimecrolimus, do they penetrate to act on the immune cells in the dermis?*

Professor Hugo: Yes, calcineurin inhibitors inhibit inflammation in the epidermis and dermis. The effect is comparable with that of mild corticosteroids, but function through a different mechanism.

MarcieMom: *The skin is also the area for synthesis of vitamin D. Is there any relationship between the sufficiency of vitamin D and normal skin functioning? And if vitamin D is required, is it best obtained from the sun or from supplements or from eating whole foods?*

Professor Hugo: There are a lot of studies on the role of vitamin D in allergy, including eczema and asthma. The results are contradictory, not convincing, but it seems that lack of vitamin D is a risk factor for allergy. Vitamin D is best obtained from the sun and from foods. Only in patients with vitamin D insufficiency, extra administration of vitamin D is indicated. Its role on eczema is very questionable.

MarcieMom: *For patients with eczema, do their skin synthesise vitamin D as one with normal skin would?*

Professor Hugo: No studies are available on this, but we assume they do.

MarcieMom: *Similarly, for a child with eczema, is he or she more susceptible to the harmful UV rays? If yes, should parents be advised to avoid direct sun, apply higher SPF sunscreen and wear protective clothing for their child?*

Professor Hugo: The answer is yes. If your child has active eczema, the sun should be avoided. If the lesions get burned by the sun, the inflammation might get worse, resulting in a flare up of eczema. If the eczema is under control (no inflammation), a little sun might have a stabilising effect (as in UV treatment in eczema, which was mainly studied in adults — no good studies in children), but be careful. The general rule is still to avoid the sun.

MarcieMom: *As the itch present in eczema will cause the patient to scratch, will such scratching damage the nerve cells on the skin and render the patient unable to feel the pain from scratching? If yes, will the patient continue to feel the itch (and not the pain from scratching), and thereby be more likely to scratch?*

Professor Hugo: This is possible, but difficult to assess and study. Studies on itch and scratching have been performed in adults, not in children. In general, different nerve cells are involved in itch, and different mechanisms of itch exist. In eczema, pain from scratching seems to be less compared to other skin diseases. In eczema, itch can be very severe and unrelated to pain from scratching.

MarcieMom: *Is the skin pH of a baby with eczema different from that without? If there is a difference, does this difference mean that babies with eczema should (i) eat foods of lower pH or (ii) use skincare products of a lower pH?*

Professor Hugo: There have been no studies on this. Moisturising seems to be the best treatment to prevent new eczema lesions. Substances that lower pH seem to be ineffective on eczema lesions.

MarcieMom: *Is there anything that can be done to improve the skin microbiota of an infant? For instance, the mother taking probiotics during pregnancy?*

Professor Hugo: There are indications that probiotics taken by the mother during pregnancy and in combination with breast feeding decrease the development of eczema. However, probiotics in formula seem to be far less effective. Our own study on probiotics in a formula, in Singaporean babies was negative. More studies are needed, but we need to realise that eczema is a complex disease. Therefore, one intervention is unlikely to have a major effect.

MarcieMom: *The Hygiene Hypothesis has been interpreted by some mothers to mean they should expose their infants to dirt, and possibly, avoid the use of anti-bacterial products. Is this recommended? I'm thinking that infants have lower immunity, and for infants with defective skin barrier, they would be even more susceptible to the penetration of irritants or allergens, or more susceptible to bacterial infection. So, should a mother take more hygiene precautions for her infant if there is a higher risk of eczema or allergy (judging from family history)?*

Professor Hugo: In theory this is correct, but the problem is that every baby is unique and needs a different degree of exposure of immune stimuli. This is very difficult to assess in a baby. However, in general, products that destroy the body's own bacteria, such as antibiotics, should be avoided and only given if necessary (in case of a bacterial infection). There have been studies showing that early administration of antibiotics increases the risk for subsequent allergy, including eczema. Hygiene precautions taken by parents seem to have little impact on the development of eczema.

MarcieMom: *The possibility of the gut microbiota having an influence on skin microbiota is very interesting. Is this anything to do with leaky gut that I often heard about?*

Professor Hugo: The gut contains the largest amount of germs, which influence the immune system. The mechanisms of the interactions between gut microbiota and immune system are still largely unknown, but have little to do with leaky gut. It is more likely that the composition of stools directly influence the skin microbiota. How much effect this has is unknown, but stools come into contact with skin, and direct contact might be the mechanism. But this needs further study.

MarcieMom: *Why is eczema patchy, with some parts of the body less affected than others?*

Professor Hugo: No idea, but local immune responses might differ according to the skin area. Also, microbiota differ according to the skin area. Finally, skin barrier features might differ. All this needs more study.

MarcieMom: *Does eczema appear in one area, improve, and then another area gets affected? If yes, why?*

Professor Hugo: Eczema is fluctuating. There is little pattern in the distribution at one time point. Usually, in time, the affected areas differ, but we have no idea why.

PART 2

Living with Eczema

CHAPTER 3

Eczema Diagnosis

Common Diagnosis Methods

When a child has a chronic rash, it may or may not be atopic dermatitis (AD) and a doctor's consultation is advised. The doctor will start by taking your child's medical history to gather useful information on the possibility of AD. The information that can assist in forming an accurate diagnosis is on:

Family History

AD is genetically determined, and a lot of genes can be involved. Therefore, there is a higher likelihood of a patient having AD if there is a family history of AD, allergic rhinitis or asthma, which are chronic diseases that are related to allergy. The risk is higher when both parents suffer from an allergic disease, or when AD is present in at least one parent.

Major genes that are involved in eczema are genes responsible for skin barrier function, such as the filaggrin (FLG) gene, and genes that are associated with allergy.

FLG is a skin barrier protein that is involved in smoothness of the skin (i.e. maintaining a spontaneous moisturised skin), and without it (i.e. null-mutation) the skin is dry and thick. However, not all children with AD have an absent FLG. FLG is merely absent in those children with severe AD, dry skin and with allergy. But there are also children with severe eczema, dry skin and allergy with normal FLG. Taken together, in all children with AD, FLG is absent in about 30%, the more severe the AD the higher the risk for a FLG deficiency. Other skin barrier proteins are now studied in AD, but, for the moment, FLG is the best studied one.

Allergy (or atopy, referring to its family occurrence) means that the child has an increased risk of developing allergic reactions to allergens, having also a genetic predisposition. However, AD can exist without allergic reactions, mainly mild AD, and allergic reactions can also be a consequence of AD.

Past Medical History

The past medical history will focus on the age of onset of the rash, the duration, the pattern (i.e. flares), on triggers, and on the existence of other allergic problems that can be associated with eczema, such as asthma, allergic rhinitis and food allergy. The age of onset of AD is very important to know. Early onset suggests a congenital skin barrier defect and the possibility of food allergy to cow's milk or hen's egg. Late onset suggests suggest no food allergy, the presence of local immune abnormalities, a house dust mite allergy or bacterial involvement as a cause.

Information on severity of the itch, on the number of hours of disrupted sleep or disruption to daily activities, will not help in coming to a diagnosis, but will give the physician an idea of the impact on the patient's quality of life and severity of AD.

Examination of the Skin

The diagnosis of AD is based on clinical examination of the skin. Usually, diagnosing AD is not difficult, but a number of other diseases always need to be excluded (see differential diagnosis), especially when AD presents with unusual features.

Itch is the most common symptom of eczema, and looking for scratch lesions is part of the clinical examination. As mentioned in Chapter 1, the lesions of AD are non-specific and made up by ichtyosis (dry skin),

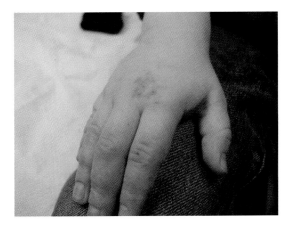

Fig. 3.1 Erythema (redness).

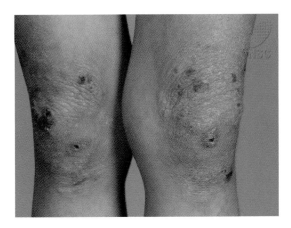

Fig. 3.2 Severe eczema in a four-year old boy with dry skin, skin interruptions (excoriations) and bacterial colonisation. (Courtesy of the National Skin Centre, Singapore.)

erythema (redness), excoriation (interruption of the skin), scratching lesions, lichenification (thickening of the skin), infected lesions (blisters, pus formation), and hypopigmentation or hyperpigmentation in old lesions.

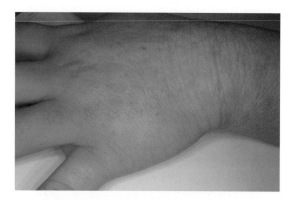

Fig. 3.3   Lichenification (thickening of skin).

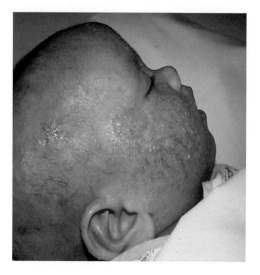

Fig. 3.4   Infected eczema on baby's face.

Differential Diagnosis of AD

A number of unrelated skin disorders can resemble eczema and have to be excluded, especially when the lesions occur in previously healthy, older children with no history of any allergic disorder. These include:

Scabies

Scabies is a contagious skin infection caused by the mite *Sarcoptes scabiei*. The mite is a tiny, and usually, not directly visible parasite, which burrows under the host's skin, causing intense itching. The infection can occur at all ages, usually affecting other members of the family. The rash is very itchy, and the body can be covered with scratch lesions. Lesions often affect the armpits, the tummy and the skin areas between fingers and toes. Treatment is specific and involves the whole family.

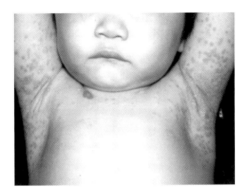

Fig. 3.5 Child with scabies.

Gianotti-Crosti syndrome

Gianotti-Crosti Syndrome is an acute to chronic (weeks to months) acrodermatitis (dermatitis of the extremities) of unknown cause, but associated with sun exposure and infections (hepatitis, infectious mononucleosis, and others). It is generally recognised as a papular (red dots) or papulo-vesicular (blisters) skin rash occurring mainly on the face and distal aspects of the four limbs. There is no specific treatment, but underlying infections have to be ruled out.

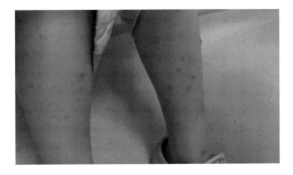

Fig. 3.6 Gianotti-Crosti syndrome.

Psoriasis

Psoriasis is rare in children, but may resemble AD. Usually, there is a positive family history. The lesions are thick, well delineated, and on normal skin.

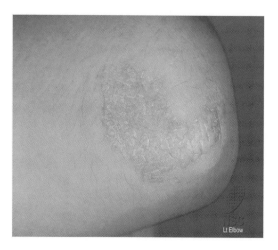

Fig. 3.7 Psoriasis. (Courtesy of the National Skin Centre, Singapore.)

Prurigo Nodularis

Prurigo nodularis resembles AD, and according to some doctors it is an expression of eczema. The nodular lesions are mainly on the extremities, and are very itchy. Secondary infections can occur.

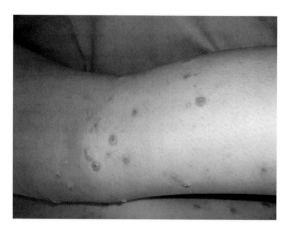

Fig. 3.8 Prurigo nodularis.

Skin infections

Skin infections can resemble AD. These are FUNGAL SKIN INFECTIONS and BED BUGS. Typically, these infections occur in previously healthy children. Therefore, in all children with a so-called sudden onset of AD, skin infections need to be excluded.

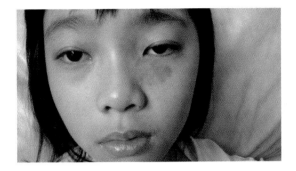

Fig. 3.9   Infection on child's face.

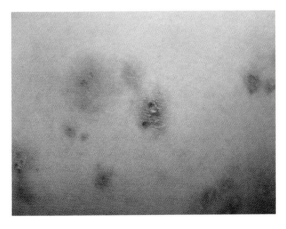

Fig. 3.10   Bed bugs.

Immune disorders

In some children with severe eczema, recurrent infections and growth retardation, an underlying immune deficiency needs to be ruled out. These immune disorders are extremely rare, but important to diagnose. Examples are Wiskott–Aldrich Syndrome and Hyper-IgE Syndrome.

Allergy Testing

Additional testing is not necessary in most children with mild AD, because the diagnosis can be made clinically. However, a few tests can be useful in children with severe AD or with frequent flare-ups. These include:

1. Allergy testing: skin prick tests (SPT) or determination of specific IgE in the blood.
2. Cultures of the skin for bacteria or viruses.

In a minority of children other tests may be indicated, especially in those with severe AD, and mainly to exclude other diseases or to diagnose the possibility of an underlying immune deficiency.

Skin prick test (SPT)

Despite progress in modern diagnostic technology, skin prick testing (SPT) is still considered as the test of choice in diagnosing allergy in children and adults. Especially in young children and infants, SPT is more sensitive than determining specific IgE. SPT is cheap, rapid, and an accurate way of identifying the causative allergens. Moreover, SPT is uncomplicated, and with practice and adherence to a few simple guidelines, it is possible to get highly reproducible results. SPT depends on the introduction of the allergen into the epidermis resulting in an IgE-mediated response, which is characterised by an immediate wheal and flare reaction. When the allergen is introduced into the skin on a previously sensitised individual, IgE molecules on the surface of a mast cell are bridged and degranulation of the mast cell occurs.

Technique

SPT is best performed on the volar or inner aspect of the forearms avoiding the flexures and the wrist areas. Under the age of three years, SPT may be more easily performed on the child's back. It is important to explain the

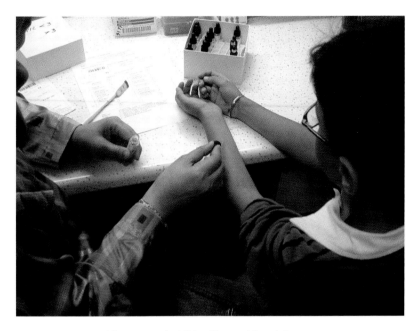

Fig. 3.11 A child taking a skin prick test.

SPT procedure to children and parents. This will lead to co-operation and a positive attitude from parents and children. A lancet with a 1 mm point is used to prick the skin through the drop. With the so-called "prick through drop" method it is unnecessary to scratch or lift the skin and no blood should be drawn. Reactions should occur within 10–15 minutes after which the results can be assessed. A positive and negative control must be included in each series of tests. The negative control solution is the diluent used to preserve the allergen extract. The positive control solution is a 1 mg/ml histamine hydrochloride solution and is used to detect hyporeactivity of the skin, including suppression by medication. Another useful positive control, especially in young children, is codeine, a mast cell degranulator, and marker of the presence of mast cells in the skin.

Interpretation of SPT results

It is important that each clinic is consistent with respect to the method it uses to report its SPT results. In general, a wheal reaction of 3 mm greater

Table 3.1   Grading of SPT

+	3 mm wheal with flare
++	3 mm to 5 mm wheal with flare
+++	> 5 mm wheal with flare
++++	> 5 mm wheal with flare and pseudopodia

than the negative control, with an appropriate histamine wheal reaction of 3 mm or more, is regarded as positive. In infants, a SPT reaction is positive when the wheal is at least ¾ of the histamine reaction. Grading of SPT may be expressed in absolute values (millimeters — centimeters), or as a percentage of the positive histamine control, or may be measured as in Table 3.1:

Usually, results of inhalant allergens are more reliable than those for foods (high number of false positive and false negative reactions, especially in children with AD). In some patients a delayed skin reaction occurs about 3–5 hours after the skin test has been performed and it is important to remind all patients to look out for these. **Dermographism** may occur as a result of the patient's skin being excessively sensitive to friction or pressure rather than to an allergen. If the patient exhibits this reaction, the negative control will also show a wheal and flare reaction. Any reading 3 mm larger than the negative control will then be read as positive. It is also important that the child is in a good clinical condition at the time of the SPT, in order to perform the test on a normally functioning immune system. Severe infections or prolonged fever may suppress the results of SPT.

Safety of SPT

Systemic reactions are extremely rare, especially in children, but may occur if the SPT is performed in a severe unstable asthmatic patient or in a pollen-sensitive patient at the height of the pollen season. Care should also be taken when testing patients with severe food allergy (such as in children with systemic reactions to peanuts) and in patients with severe drug allergy. Therefore, it is recommended to have emergency resuscitative equipment available.

Factors influencing SPT

All **medications containing antihistamine** need to be stopped prior to testing as they effectively block the wheal and flare reaction. In general, it is recommended to stop all anti-histamines for three to seven days before SPT.

Other conditions affecting results of SPT

1. Infants and young children may have low skin reactivity (due to low numbers of mast cells in the skin), and interpretation of SPT results is more difficult.
2. Severe eczema and old eczema lesions may cause hyporeactivity of the skin, because of intensive subcutaneous scaring of the skin.
3. Incorrect technique and loss of potency of allergy solutions due to incorrect or prolonged storage.

SPT is safe, simple and cheap, with immediate reproducible results available to the clinician. In conjunction with the case history and clinical findings, it still remains the key diagnostic tool in childhood allergic diseases.

Patch Test

In children there is little data on the value of patch tests. Therefore, patch testing is almost never used as a diagnostic test in AD. More literature is available in adults, and patch testing can be used in the diagnosis of contact eczema. Its role in AD is still very controversial, both in adults and children, and patch testing should not be used in diagnosing AD.

A patch test is usually used for testing a delayed immune response, the so-called type IV immune response in which T-lymphocytes are the major player. It can also be used to differentiate irritant contact dermatitis from allergic contact dermatitis, mainly in adults, and no data is available in children.

Total IgE and Allergen-specific IgE Blood Test

IgE is the antibody that is responsible for allergic reactions. Determining allergen-specific IgE in the blood of the patient is therefore of value in diagnosing the existence of allergy. Several methods to determine IgE in serum (blood) have been developed. The old methods showed little sensitivity and specificity, but with the new methods, determination of specific IgE is highly reliable, showing good sensitivity (= detection of low concentrations) and specificity (= few false positive results).

Therefore, determination of **antigen-specific IgE** is a better method than the determination of total IgE to diagnose allergy, and its value is similar to skin prick testing. Nowadays, there are more than 400 characterised allergens available for *in vitro* diagnostic tests and several useful methodologies for specific IgE determination. Specific IgE results obtained with the different methods vary significantly, with absolute agreement in about 55–65% of the cases. The specificity of the anti-IgE antibody used in the assay is of critical importance because any contaminant antibody can render unspecific results. On the other hand, it must be pointed out that there is a compromise between specificity and sensitivity, such that an increase in the sensitivity of a technique leads to a decrease in its specificity. It cannot be said that there is one method which is better than the others; it is better to examine them individually, allergen by allergen. Thus, specific IgE determination varies depending on the type of allergen. In general terms, for inhalant allergens, specificity and sensitivity of the methods are within the range of 85–95%, but these values (especially the specificity) decrease in the case of food allergens, and they are still lower when the allergen is a beta-lactam antibiotic. There is a good correlation between clinical history and specific IgE against inhalant allergens, and a lower correlation in the case of food allergens. Due to the fact that most food allergens are not standardised, the definitive diagnosis of food hypersensitivity is still achieved by means of double-blind placebo-controlled provocation tests.

The first immunometric assay, called the radioallergosorbent test (RAST), was developed in 1967. It involved adding the patient's serum to the allergen disc filled with suspected allergens. Should the serum contain IgE antibodies specific to the suspected allergen, these antibodies will bind themselves to the allergen. Anti-human IgE antibody is then added to the disc, which will bind specifically with the IgE antibody that has already bound with the allergen. The unbound antibody is then washed away, and

The RAST test

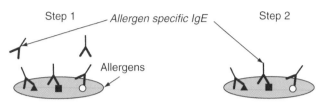

Step 1 — Allergen specific IgE — Step 2

The serum sample is incubated with an allergen disc. During this step, IgE molecules with specificities for the various allergenic components bind to the allergen disc.

Proteins non-specifically bound are washed away with a buffer containing detergent. Only specifically bound IgE remains on the disc.

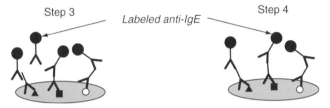

Step 3 — Labeled anti-IgE — Step 4

The disc is incubated with labeled anti-human IgE antibody, which binds specifically to the IgE on the disc. The amount of labeled antibody bound is directly proportional to the amount of IgE present on the disc.

Unbound antibody is washed away with buffer containing detergent.

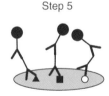

Step 5

Specific IgE is quantitated either through the reaction of labeled antibody with an enzyme substrate (EIA), or by counting radioactivity (RAST).

Fig. 3.12 RAST test.

the remaining specific IgE can be quantified. A more current blood test is known as the CAP-FEIA (or immunoCAP) test, where a cellulose sponge is activated and able to bind large amounts of allergens, thereby increasing the sensitivity of the test. It may be prescribed in certain instances such as comparing the scores to charts to determine the risk of allergic reaction or for supervising if the child has possibly outgrown a certain food allergy. The other type of blood test is the enzyme-linked immunosorbent essay (ELISA, or EIA), which uses a nonradioactive signal via enzyme which is linked to specific antibody, and the presence of an allergy detected through the change in color of the solution.

Remarks on total IgE

While specific IgE is directed against specific allergens, total IgE is the sum of all IgE present in the blood, not only against allergens, but also against micro-organisms, such as viruses or parasites. The value of determining total IgE, via radioimmunosorbent test (RIST), in diagnosing allergy is *limited*, as it only gives an idea about the potential of the patient to produce IgE. Although many allergic patients have a raised total IgE, this can also be found in non-allergic patients, for instance, in children after viral or parasitic infections. Therefore, total IgE determination is considered a method for the screening of allergic diseases, though its actual value is controversial because normal values of total IgE do not exclude the existence of an allergic disease, and high values of total IgE are not specific of allergy by itself.

Oral Food Challenge

The oral food challenge is still the gold standard to determine if a food allergy exists and may be suggested by the physician in instances where the results of the skin prick test, IgE blood test and the patient's observations do not corroborate. The best type of oral food challenge is the double-blind, placebo-controlled challenge (DBPCC), in which doctor and patient are blinded to the food that is administrated. It is also useful to establish if the child has "outgrown" his allergy. However, an oral food challenge is seldom prescribed by the physician due to the length of time and costs involved.

The oral food challenge is carried out in the hospital and involves putting the patient under observation while increasing the quantities of the food to the child. It is important to have it conducted in a hospital where an allergic reaction can be addressed before it progresses to a severe, life-threatening reaction, such as an anaphylactic reaction or anaphylactic shock. Oral challenges should never be carried out at home!

A note on allergy tests

It is worthwhile to mention here that SPT and blood tests are never 100% accurate: A positive result can be noted but the patient does not exhibit any sign of allergic reaction or it is also possible for the patient to show signs of an allergic reaction with negative allergy tests results. While the tests are not foolproof, they remain the most useful diagnostic tools and a practical reference point for patients to manage their eczema, through the elimination or minimisation of triggers of eczema flare-ups.

Skin Biopsy

Skin biopsy is hardly used in children, and only used when the eczema is severe and has not responded to previous treatments. Indications for a skin

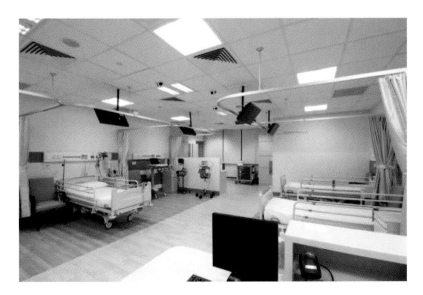

Fig. 3.13 Facilities for oral provocation tests at the Department of Paediatrics, National University Hospital, Singapore.

biopsy are to rule out other severe underlying diseases, and to culture for fungi or yeasts in patients with therapy-resistant eczema.

Different methods are used to obtain a skin sample. These include: a shave biopsy, punch biopsy, excisional biopsy, and incisional biopsy. The choice of skin biopsy will depend on the type of skin lesion.

Patient's Observations

The physician will also gather information from the parents or the patient on his/her own observations, relating to environmental or food triggers. Certain triggers are more prevalent for certain age groups, but generally for all, detergents and soaps, sweat, heat, low humidity (in winter), "prickly" non-cotton clothing, stress and sudden temperature changes can induce flare-ups.

In infants, foods such as egg, cow's milk, soy and wheat are more likely to trigger an eczema flare-up than in older children, where house dust mites are a more common allergen. However, before starting a diet in a child with AD it is recommended to have a good and specific diagnosis. Identifying foods as a trigger for eczema is extremely difficult in day-to-day life, and often parents identify the wrong foods. Parents may also observe worsening skin rash for the child during a fever or cold. The symptoms of AD can be aggravated during periods of fluctuating hormones, such as puberty and menopause. Pregnant women may also observe a flare-up of their eczema, likewise for some women during certain periods of their menstrual cycle.

Diagnostic Criteria for AD

The diagnosis of AD is usually straightforward. In difficult cases criteria can be used. There are numerous diagnostic criteria for AD, among which are Hanifin and Rajka (1980), UK Diagnostic (1994), Schultz-Larsen (1992), Diepgen (1996), Kang and Tian (1989), Lillehammer (1994) and by International Study of Asthma and Allergies in Childhood (ISAAC) (1995).

Hanifin and Rajka were the first to set out diagnostic criteria, listing a total of four major and 23 minor criteria, and AD is diagnosed should there be three major and three minor criteria present.

The four major criteria are:

1. Pruritus
2. Flexural lichenification or linearity in adults or rashes on the face and flexural areas in children
3. Chronic dermatitis
4. Personal or family history of atopy

The American Academy of Dermatology has also suggested criteria for diagnosis for AD that is classified into essential, important and associated features. Essential features are pruritus and eczematous changes that are acute, subacute or chronic, and when present are sufficient to diagnose AD. Important features are the onset of AD at an early stage, atopy and xerosis, while associated features include icthyosis, atypical vascular responses, lichenification, ocular/periorbital changes and perioral/periauricular lesions.

Assessment of the severity of AD

The severity of AD can be assessed, and at the same time a diagnosis is made by using the scoring system SCORAD (Scoring Atopic Dermatitis). This can be used to assess the improvement of AD in the follow-up consultation.

Mom Asks, Doc Answers!

MarcieMom: *Visiting a doctor may cause some anxiety for patients, particularly for parents who are uncertain of what to expect and how to effectively communicate their child's skin condition. I know when I came to see you, I was armed with a detailed food diary and a list of suspected food allergens but the skin prick test returned negative results for all the common food allergens! As a physician, what information do you think it is good for the patient to think through to communicate to you at the first consultation?*

Professor Hugo: The doctor will ask many questions. These include: questions on onset, duration, itch, possible triggers and the existence of other allergic disorders, such as asthma or allergic rhinitis. It is important to know whether there is a positive family history of eczema and if there are obvious triggers — not suspected triggers. To have a good idea about previous eczema treatments is important.

MarcieMom: *Does family history include food allergy of family members?*

Professor Hugo: Yes, all allergic reactions, including food allergy, allergic asthma, allergic rhinitis, point to the existence of an allergic constitution, hereby increasing the risk of allergy in the offspring.

MarcieMom: *Do you have any statistics relating to the likelihood of a child getting AD should one or both parents or siblings have AD?*

Professor Hugo: Usually eczema runs in the family, but new sporadic cases do occur. The more allergies running in the family, the higher the risk for eczema or for another allergic disease. When both parents are allergic or both parents have eczema, the risk is very high, almost 80% to 90%.

MarcieMom: *Is maternal eczema the strongest predictor of eczema in the child?*

Professor Hugo: Yes, it is. However, we are talking about atopic dermatitis. In cases of contact dermatitis the risk is lower.

MarcieMom: *If more than one person has eczema in the family, do they all react to the same triggers?*

Professor Hugo: Not necessary. Hereditary of eczema is complex and only partially understood. Usually, triggers are age-related and also dependent on the environment. In one family with different members suffering from eczema, totally different triggers can be present in the different family members.

MarcieMom: *Are airborne allergens (other than house dust mites) and exposure to irritants associated with a late onset of eczema?*

Professor Hugo: This is possible, especially for pollen. The role of irritants in atopic dermatitis is far less clear. However, irritants can be involved in contact dermatitis.

MarcieMom: *The patient will not be able to identify whether the skin rash is AD, irritant contact dermatitis, allergic contact dermatitis or other skin diseases. As such, when enquiring on the patient's medical history, the skin rash that first occurred may or may not be the same skin disease that he/she is experiencing. Does this significantly affect an accurate diagnosis of AD? Also, would it help in your diagnosis if a patient takes photographs of their previous skin rash?*

Professor Hugo: Photographs are very useful. Usually, children only suffer from one skin disease, and the occurrence of different types of eczema in one child is rare. However, eczema by itself is dynamic, from mild to severe and vice versa, dependent on triggers, superimposed infection, and treatments.

MarcieMom: *Is dry skin in a newborn apparent?*

Professor Hugo: Not always. A child with severe eczema may have perfect skin at birth. When the skin is obviously dry at birth there is a higher risk that the child will develop eczema.

MarcieMom: *There are common skin conditions such as baby/neonatal acne that do not warrant a doctor's consultation and will resolve on its own. When should a parent suspect eczema and seek a doctor's consultation?*

Professor Hugo: Mainly when the baby is uncomfortable or when the skin is dry or covered with red patches. In general, if a parent feels there is something wrong with the baby's skin, it is safer to see a doctor.

MarcieMom: *Depending on the country that the patient resides in, he/she may have to wait a certain period for a consultation or an allergy test. It is not uncommon to see pictures of skin rashes posted on forums asking if anyone thinks it is eczema. I'm wondering if there exists a possibility for the diagnosis of AD to be done without a face-to-face consultation.*

Professor Hugo: It is difficult, as other diseases can be present. I advise to ask for a doctor's help if your child's skin is abnormal. Don't start treating your child without a good diagnosis, or you might do something wrong.

MarcieMom: *In Singapore, when children develop rashes, it's sometimes referred to as "heat rash" which some take to mean rashes due to the hot weather in Singapore. Is heat rash actually eczema triggered by heat?*

Professor Hugo: Children with eczema are more sensitive to heat, causing flare-up of the eczema. Some other conditions of sensitive skin, such as urticaria or dermographism, may also flare-up due to heat. However, heat rash by itself is not a good diagnosis, and a reason for it needs to be established.

MarcieMom: *What are the symptoms of AD on the eyelids? Also for young children that scratch their eyelids frequently, what are the possible negative impacts to the eyelid and to the eye?*

Professor Hugo: The symptoms are the same as for other parts of the skin. When scratching the eyes there is a risk for eye infection, but usually eczema does not affect the eye, only the surrounding skin.

MarcieMom: *As a mother to a lovely girl, I hope that eczema will not affect her appearance as she grows older. Can a child's skin be permanently damaged?*

Professor Hugo: Yes, it can, especially when the eczema is untreated, resulting in infection of the skin. This can lead to hyperpigmentation, hypopigmentation and scarring lesions of the skin. My advice: Treat all red patches as soon as possible and keep the bacteria on the skin low, by regular swimming in chlorinated water or by using antiseptics (antibiotics should be avoided, and soap has little to no effect on skin bacteria).

MarcieMom: *Puberty presents a time of hormonal change for teenagers. How does this affect the skin? Is there a difference between the symptoms of eczema in teenage males and females?*

Professor Hugo: Usually, puberty has a suppressing effect upon eczema and upon allergy. A lot of children get better during puberty. In some, however, the symptoms can persist. Usually more boys grow out of allergy, as compared to girls, but exact data on eczema are not available. Most studies were done in adolescents with asthma.

MarcieMom: *Is hand eczema more commonly seen in adults, and why?*

Professor Hugo: Yes, but it is not an allergic eczema, but mainly a contact eczema, due to irritants (soaps, chemicals), and linked to daily working activities.

MarcieMom: *I understand that every individual has his own skin microbial profile. For the elderly, is there any condition (say diabetes) that alters the patient's microbial profile and increase the likelihood of skin diseases?*

Professor Hugo: Every disease and a lot of treatments, such as antibiotics, may affect the skin microbiota. The risk to develop eczema in elderly is low. Skin infections occur more in elderly people suffering from diabetes.

MarcieMom: *In my experience moderating and participating in eczema forums, I have come across numerous accounts of patients whose doctors did not prescribe an allergy test. Should a patient request for an allergy test? Also, can a patient obtain an allergy test without a doctor's consultation? Is that recommended?*

Professor Hugo: Allergy testing is not recommended for all children with eczema, but only for those with severe eczema unresponsive to standard treatment. In those children, an underlying allergy needs to be excluded. In theory, parents can get an allergy test for their child without a doctor's consult, but parents usually don't know which test and which allergens to screen for. Furthermore, an allergy test needs an appropriate interpretation, which can only be given by a specialist in allergy.

MarcieMom: *Is there any study on the accuracies of the skin prick test in children and adults? Can you share with us some of the data?*

Professor Hugo: There have been many studies over many years on the SPT. In short, the SPT is the best test to diagnose allergy in most children and adults. Exceptions are those patients in whom a SPT cannot be performed for various reasons.

MarcieMom: *I understand that the skin prick test is fairly accurate in determining what is not an allergen than it is in predicting what is an allergen. Is that correct?*

Professor Hugo: Both are correct. You are referring to sensitivity and specificity. The SPT shows the presence or absence of allergy, without answering whether this allergy is involved in the symptoms.

MarcieMom: *Therefore, should a parent introduce the allergen tested positive but which he/she suspect is a false positive on their own? Is there a best practice method of introducing the allergen systematically that will help the parent confirm if a possible allergen is indeed triggering the child's eczema?*

Professor Hugo: When a SPT is positive, one should avoid the allergen. It can be dangerous if parents start experimenting with allergens. The best tactic is avoidance. Introduction can lead to tolerance, I agree, but also to worsening of the allergy. Provocation with an allergen should be done according to the doctor's advice and in a hospital setting.

MarcieMom: *While the skin prick test is a faster, more reliable and cheaper option than the blood test, I have heard of parents avoiding it because the name "skin prick" test sounds like it would be traumatising for the child. What do you do in your practice to encourage fearful parents to let their children take the SPT?*

Professor Hugo: A good SPT, performed by an experienced person, should be painless. In our department we say that a SPT should be associated with no blood and no cry, even in infants.

MarcieMom: *In a skin prick test, the size and appearance of the wheal is analysed to determine if there is an allergy. What would be the circumstances whereby the results of the tests will prompt you to request for a retest or for a different type of allergy test?*

Professor Hugo: Sometimes it can be difficult to interpret a SPT, especially in young children, at the onset of an allergy. Moreover, allergy in young children is very dynamic. In case of doubt, we usually recommend to repeat the SPT after six months.

MarcieMom: *Patients may wrongly assume that the size of the wheal is an indication of the severity of the allergic reaction. Is it a common practice not to let patient know which wheal is for which allergen (to prevent the patient from misinterpreting it on his/her own)?*

Professor Hugo: No, we show the results to the parents. Severity of a SPT does not mean that the disease will be more severe. It only points to a higher risk for involvement of allergy into the symptoms.

MarcieMom: *What are the common types of antihistamines and medication that the patient should avoid prior to a skin prick test?*

Professor Hugo: All antihistamines should be avoided for at least 3 days, preferably for 3 to 7 days. All other medication can be continued.

MarcieMom: *Does the SPT cause sensitisation to the allergen?*

Professor Hugo: No, this has never been shown. SPT is considered safe and accurate.

MarcieMom: *Why are testing certain foods such as egg, cow's milk and peanut sufficient in a skin prick test? How do physicians know that no common food allergen has been left out in the test?*

Professor Hugo: It's all about knowledge of which foods are involved in eczema, according to age. In infants the most common food involved in eczema is hen's egg, followed by cow's milk, wheat and soy. In older children other foods can be involved, but food allergy as a trigger of eczema becomes less common in older children.

MarcieMom: *What is the accuracy of a patch test?*

Professor Hugo: No good data is available in children. We don't use patch testing in children with eczema.

MarcieMom: *How does the patch test administered by the physician differ from the "patch test" a patient tries on her own (by applying a small amount of the product onto a small area of skin and observing the reaction (if any))?*

Professor Hugo: All tests should be standardised. If you use the wrong concentration of an allergen, a test can result in a false positive or false negative. I don't recommend testing your own child with crude food extracts. It will give you the wrong information and can be dangerous.

MarcieMom: *What is the accuracy of IgE blood test?*

Professor Hugo: It is specific, but less sensitive then a SPT, resulting in more false negative results.

MarcieMom: *How do you normally advise a patient whose child is tested allergic to many food groups? Would excluding all of the foods be appropriate? Or should there be a planned elimination diet where there is a systematic and reliable way of monitoring if certain foods can be added back to the diet, and how? What is a suitable time frame to do so without compromising the nutrition that a growing child needs?*

Professor Hugo: Many food allergies in one patient are very unusual. Most children are allergic to one or two foods, usually to eggs and cow's milk. I ask to avoid eggs and to replace cow's milk by another type of milk, usually soy or an hypoallergenic (HA)-milk. Some children allergic to peanuts have to avoid all nuts. Other common allergies are seafood and fish, which also need to be avoided. Introducing or re-introducing a food needs to be done according to the type of food, the severity of the allergy and the disease status of the child. Individual advice needs to be given, no general rules. Knowledge about long-term evolution of a specific food allergy is necessary. Some food allergies are temporarily (such as cow's milk or egg), others are more persistent (peanut, seafood).

MarcieMom: *Due to false positives from the results of an IgE blood test, parents may have excluded certain foods from the diet of a growing child with no obvious improvement in the skin condition. Unfortunately, eczema comes and goes and it is difficult for the parent to directly relate certain food eliminations with the skin's appearance. Does a parent need to consult a doctor before adding the tested positive foods back to the child's diet?*

Professor Hugo: Yes, don't introduce the food by yourself at home. This can be dangerous. Parents need to understand that a diet by itself will not cure eczema, only eliminate a food trigger. Eczema is complex, and mainly a skin barrier disease. Other non-specific triggers (stress, heat, sweat) are usually present, especially in children with severe eczema. Food is only one of the many triggers, but avoidable.

MarcieMom: *Suppose a patient has undergone both a skin prick test and IgE blood test and the results differ between the two tests. Should the patient avoid an allergen as long as it is tested positive in one of the tests or only avoid an allergen that is tested positive in both sets of tests? How would a physician normally interpret differing test results and advise the patient?*

Professor Hugo: It is all about interpretation of test results and taking no risks. In case of doubt, and if the symptoms are severe and persist, a provocation test can bring the solution. In most children with eczema, interpretation is straightforward.

MarcieMom: *Can the IgE blood test be used to monitor the outgrowing of a child's allergy?*

Professor Hugo: IgE can be used, especially in cases of peanut allergy. For most other allergies, and knowing the natural evolution of an allergy, monitoring by IgE is not necessary. A repeat SPT can also be used, especially in young children who are allergic to cow's milk or eggs.

MarcieMom: *I also understand that IgG blood test is used to determine food sensitivities. Can you explain the IgG blood test, its accuracy and when do you think a patient ought to take this test?*

Professor Hugo: An IgG test shows contact with the allergen. All of us have IgG towards the food that we eat. IgG has absolutely no value in the diagnosis of allergy.

MarcieMom: *Will excluding a food or avoiding an environmental allergen lead to the patient having a longer-term allergy to it, versus one who systematically adds back the allergen?*

Professor Hugo: No, the general rule is to avoid the allergen to which the child is allergic, and not to test it yourself as a parent.

MarcieMom: *Is there a national guideline or international guideline on what age a child is before he/she can start allergy testing?*

Professor Hugo: Allergy can be tested at all ages, even in newborns. The thing is that sensitisation can take some time. Therefore, allergy testing is rarely indicated in very young infants, but in theory can be performed.

MarcieMom: *How often or under what circumstances would you suggest for a child to retake the allergy test?*

Professor Hugo: This varies individually, depending on the evolution of the allergy and the type of allergy. Sometimes we retest every year, sometimes never again.

MarcieMom: *Since allergy tests may not be accurate for infants, how would a parent know which are the allergens? Are there common allergens and irritants that trigger eczema flare-ups for infants and how can a parent observe if they are applicable for the child?*

Professor Hugo: Allergy tests can be done at all ages, but usually are not commonly indicated in young children. A general rule: If an allergy is involved in the symptoms of the child, the allergy will show in SPT or in IgE. It is difficult for parents to observe correctly on their own what triggers the eczema, especially for food that is given frequently.

MarcieMom: *Does an oral food challenge work if the food allergy is not an immediate reaction?*

Professor Hugo: Yes, but it is more difficult to interpret as the reaction can occur after an interval (hours to a few days). In general, oral food challenges are to document immediate allergic reactions, type I (IgE-mediated).

MarcieMom: *When will a skin biopsy be recommended for a child?*

Professor Hugo: Almost never, and is certainly not routine in children with eczema! I only did a few in my long career. This was to exclude another severe disease.

MarcieMom: *Given that there are often bacteria and fungi on the infected eczema skin, should a biopsy be requested by the patient in order to know what bacteria and fungi are present so there is less trial and error in the prescription of anti-bacterial and anti-fungal topical creams?*

Professor Hugo: Skin cultures for bacteria, viruses or fungi can be performed without the need of a biopsy. Culturing is non-invasive. Never request for a skin biopsy!

MarcieMom: *In your experience, how reliable are patients' observations in relation to what is triggering his/her eczema? Is there a certain allergen or irritant that a patient usually observes accurately? Conversely, is there a certain allergen group that a patient usually observes inaccurately? And why do you think it is so?*

Professor Hugo: Most parents fail to identify the triggers of their child's eczema, or come up with lists that are non-reliable. Don't forget that eczema is a chronic disease, needing a chronic or regular trigger. This is very difficult to identify, especially when a house dust mite allergy is involved, which can mimic multiple food allergies.

MarcieMom: *In your practice, do you adopt a certain diagnostic criteria and check every one of the criteria before providing a diagnosis? I read that physicians seldom do that due to it being time-consuming, with little value added to the diagnosis. Why is this so?*

Professor Hugo: In most cases, eczema is not a difficult diagnosis. Some cases are difficult, and in these children we check criteria.

MarcieMom: *In terms of assessing the severity of the eczema, is there a standard way to communicate the severity of eczema between physicians?*

Professor Hugo: SCORAD is widely used to assess the severity. Sometimes we distinguish mild, moderate and severe eczema, which also gives a good idea on how to treat the child.

MarcieMom: *In terms of diagnosis and assessment of the applicable allergens and irritants, does switching physicians affect the accuracy of the diagnosis and ascertainment of the allergens?*

Professor Hugo: You go to and like whatever doctor who helps you. If not, you go to another.

CHAPTER 4

Triggers for Eczema

Understanding Triggers

Eczema is a chronic condition, and while there is no cure, it can be controlled. Part of an effective management approach requires identifying triggers for eczema, in order for the patient to avoid or minimise contact with the triggers to reduce instances of eczema flare-ups.

Triggers can be broadly classified into allergic triggers and non-allergic triggers. Allergic triggers include food and inhaled allergens, inducing an IgE-mediated (allergic) immune response, resulting in an inflammation of the skin. Non-allergic triggers include contact allergens, inducing inflammation (i.e. contact eczema) via a delayed immune response (type IV immune response — see below), usually without the involvement of IgE (non-IgE-mediated). Other non-allergic triggers (where IgE is not involved) induce skin inflammation mainly via irritation, which is direct triggering of inflammation. Non-allergic triggers can be further classified as originating from the person (endogenous) or from external sources (exogenous). Atopic dermatitis is mainly triggered by allergic triggers, while contact dermatitis and non-allergic eczema are triggered by non-allergic triggers. The triggers in seborrhoeic eczema are still unknown.

Allergens and the Hypersensitive Reaction

Allergens trigger an IgE-mediated immune response (type I immune response or reaction), inducing inflammation in those subjects who are allergic to them, but are harmless for non-allergic persons. Allergens belong to the large group of foreign proteins, also called antigens. According to

69

Table 4.1   Triggers

Allergic Triggers	
Food allergen	Egg, milk, wheat, soy, peanut (others are less common)
Inhaled allergen	Outdoor allergens (pollen), indoor allergens (house dust mite, cockroach, pet, mold)
Non-Allergic Triggers	
Endogenous	Psychological factors (stress and sleep deprivation)
	Infections (fever)
	Hormonal changes (puberty and pregnancy)
Exogenous	Irritant substances (soap, fragrance, detergent, wool, perspiration, hot water, etc)
	Heat
	Cold climate
	Pollutants
	Mechanical irritation
	Alcohol
Contact allergens (involved in contact eczema)	Plant, dye, nickel, leather, latex, and many others (mainly in adults, less common in children)
Bacterial colonisation	

Table 4.2   Hypersensitivity Reactions

Types of hypersensitivity reactions	
Type I reactions	Immediate hypersensitivity reactions
Type II reactions	Cytotoxic hypersensitivity reactions
Type III reactions	Immune-complex reactions
Type IV reactions	Delayed hypersensitivity reactions, cell-mediated immunity

Gell and Coombs, four types of immune responses can be distinguished in the human body (Table 4.2). Allergic reactions are type I responses, subsequently causing eczema in a secondary phase, through the induction of inflammation. Type IV reactions are reactions of the delayed type, causing inflammation without IgE involvement. Type IV reactions are usually involved in contact eczema. Type II and Type III immune reactions are usually not involved in eczema or in allergic reactions.

Other classifications of immune reactions have been proposed, but are less useful here. Every child has his or her own triggers, and the role of the physician is to identify those triggers.

The sensitisation process

An allergic reaction starts with sensitisation. This is the phase in which the allergen induces an immune response, being the production of IgE.

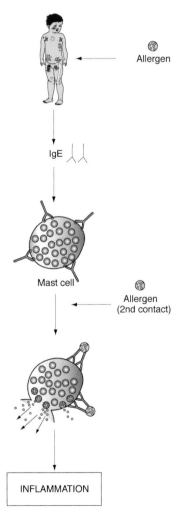

Fig. 4.1 Illustration of IgE-mediated immune response.

Antigen-specific IgE binds itself to the membrane of a number of cells, including mast cells, basophils, monocytes, and Langerhans cells. Subsequent re-exposure to the same allergen, in a sensitised person, results in the binding of the allergen to the IgE on different cells, resulting in cell activation, degranulation of different activating substances from cells, attraction of other cells, and finally in a clinical inflammatory reaction.

Food Allergens

Food allergens are proteins in foods or their derivatives that are able to induce allergic reactions in persons allergic to that food. The role of food allergy in eczema is greater in infants compared to adults, and a number of children can "outgrow" their food allergy. The prevalence of food allergy in children is between 5% and 8% and is higher in young children. Food allergy is also more common in young children with severe eczema than in those with mild eczema. In infants with severe AD, food allergy can be involved in more than 70% of them (in some studies up to 90%).

Taking together the results from different studies, it has been shown that food allergy can play a role in AD. Most positive reactions to food occur in young children with severe types of AD. However, only a limited number of foods are involved in AD. These include: eggs, cow's milk, soy, and wheat.

Table 4.3   Most Common Food Allergies in Children in Asia

INFANTS	PRESCHOOLERS	OLDER CHILDREN
— cow's milk	— cow's milk	— peanut
— eggs	— eggs	— tree nuts
— wheat	— peanut	— fish
— soy	— tree nuts	— shellfish
	— fish	— sesame
	— shellfish	— fruits
	— sesame	— bird's nest
	— fruits	
	— bird's nest	

Food Allergy (FA) in Eczema

Recent studies have shown that different situations of food allergy can exist in eczema. Undoubtedly, certain foods can induce eczema, especially in infants (eggs, milk). However, it has now been shown that eczema can also induce food allergy, mainly through transcutaneous sensitisation. This was shown mainly in children with a filaggrin-deficiency and for peanuts. Once the food allergy occurs, eczema can get worse and becomes persistent. However, eczema and food allergy can exist concomitantly without influencing each other in a number of children. Therefore, it is now accepted that different situations can exist. For each child, the impact of food on eczema has to be determined.

Briefly, the following situations are now recognised:

1. FA and AD co-exist without influencing each other
2. FA can trigger eczema
3. Eczema can induce food allergy

Food allergy mainly occurs early in life, and in eczema, a lot of children can outgrow their food allergy. This is the case for food allergy against cow's milk, eggs, soy, and wheat. However, outgrowing a food allergy doesn't mean outgrowing eczema. House dust mite allergy can develop in allergic children (usually during preschool age) and is able to maintain eczema. Therefore, it is important that the individual triggers of eczema are identified, and if the eczema persists, repeated testing is advised.

Determining a Food Allergy

As covered in Chapter 3, allergy tests such as a skin prick test and the determination of allergen-specific IgE blood test are available. The presence of IgE (i.e. positive blood test or a positive skin prick test) does not mean that the food is involved in eczema, as the food allergy can have no impact on eczema (i.e. an epiphenomenon) or can be a consequence of the eczema. False positive and false negative results do exist. The gold standard for determining whether a specific food is involved in eczema is the oral-food challenge carried out under double-blind, placebo-controlled conditions (DBPCC). Once an allergy is confirmed by the physician, the food ought to be avoided and not be re-introduced without consulting the physician. Sometimes a test diet can be used as a diagnostic tool.

Symptoms of Food Allergy

While eczema can be an expression of food allergy, especially in young children, other symptoms of food allergy, ranging from mild to severe, have been described. These include:

— Itching or swelling or tingling of lips or mouth or face.
— Hives or welts.
— Abdominal cramps and pains.
— Vomiting.
— Diarrhea.
— Swelling of tongue.
— Wheezing or coughing.
— Dizziness or fainting.
— Paleness.
— Shortness of breath (tightening of airway).
— Shock or drop in blood pressure (anaphylactic shock).

Symptoms can occur within a few minutes to hours after contact with the food (ingestion, inhaling, touching). Patients and caregivers of children must be instructed and prepared to manage the symptoms, and training on administration of epinephrine is especially recommended. Medical alert bracelets or necklaces can also be worn by the child so that the type of allergy, personal identification, details and instruction on administration of epinephrine, are available should the allergic reaction result in collapse or difficulty in speech.

Exercise-induced Food Allergy

Certain food allergies can be induced by exercise, whereby the person experiences an allergic reaction after eating the food and exercising. This can be avoided by not eating the suspected food up to 24 hours before exercising. Foods that have been identified to cause this type of reaction include seafood and wheat.

Cross-reactivity in Food Allergies

Cross-reactivity refers to the ability of the immune system to recognise similar allergens that are present in different food or inhalant allergens. For instance, a person with an allergic reaction to shrimp may also be allergic to lobster or crab or a child allergic to cow's milk is also allergic to goat's milk. Cross-reactivity reactions between food allergens and inhalant allergens have been described too, such as cross-reactivity between grass pollen and vegetables and fruits, or between ragweed pollen and melon or birch pollen and apple or other fruit allergens (labelled as Oral Allergy Syndrome = OAS). In Singapore, cross-reactivity between house dust mite and seafood has been described, due to the allergen tropomyosin, present in house dust mites and seafood.

Distinguishing Food Allergy from Food Intolerance

Unlike food allergy, food intolerance does not involve the immune system but may be confused with food allergy as there are similar symptoms such as nausea, abdominal pain, vomiting and diarrhea. Food intolerance where the person has a non-immunological (including non-IgE) mediated food hypersensitivity may present itself after consuming larger quantities of the food. In contrast, food allergy occurs after consuming little amounts. A common food intolerance is that to lactose (milk sugar), which is related to the inability to digest lactose, and therefore leads to gas production, abdominal pain or diarrhea. This is due to a deficiency of the enzyme lactase. Other food intolerances are to gluten, sulfites, and monosodium glutamate (MSG). Moreover, food intolerance can also occur because the food contains toxins or is infected (food poisoning).

A note on the elimination diet

An elimination diet involves not eating the suspected foods for a few weeks (at the direction of the physician), then adding back the foods one at a time to observe which food is triggering hypersensitive reactions. Should there be a hypersensitive reaction, the doctor may request that the suspected food be avoided. However, this may not be accurate as the reaction observed by the patient may not have been triggered by food but by environmental or endogenous factors such as stress. The elimination diet is also not safe if the hypersensitive reaction is severe, such as an anaphylaxis reaction. Parents should not implement it without medical advice. Alternative food substitutes should be consumed as a replacement for the eliminated foods, and the elimination diet should not be carried out on an ongoing basis to avoid nutrition deficiency.

A note on food labels

In the United States, the Food and Drug Administration (FDA) requires manufacturers to list the eight most common ingredients that trigger food allergies, namely milk, eggs, peanuts, tree nuts, fish, shellfish, soy, and wheat. In Singapore, there is a requirement to declare foods and ingredients known to cause hypersensitivity via either the statement of ingredients or the "contains" statement. The eight types of food under this requirement are cereals containing gluten, crustacean, eggs, fish, peanut, soybeans, milk, tree nuts and sulphites in concentrates of 10 mg/kg or more. Parents of children with food allergy should be instructed to read food labels.

Inhaled Allergens

In a number of studies, older children with AD, beyond the age of three years, are observed to have positive reactions (skin prick test and/or specific IgE) to a number of inhaled allergens. Usually, an allergy to an inhaled allergen does not occur during the first two years of life. The exact roles of these allergic reactions in AD are still a matter of debate and are not accepted as involved in AD by every researcher. The common inhaled allergens are house dust mites, pet dander, mold, cockroach antigens, and pollen. Usually these inhaled allergens are involved in respiratory diseases, such as asthma, hay fever or allergic rhinitis.

House Dust Mites

House dust mite is a common inhaled allergen, and house dust mites thrive in the home environment due to a combination of (i) room temperature, (ii) humid environment, and (iii) human dead skin, which serves as their food source. There are many species of house dust mites, but allergic symptoms are mainly (but not exclusively) induced by three species: *Dermatophagoides pteronyssinus*, *Dermatophagoides farinae*, and *Blomia tropicalis*, the latter being a common mite in tropical areas, such as Singapore.

There are also different allergens within the dust mite droppings, which vary in size, and therefore some tend to be more airborne than others, *versus* the larger allergen particles that tend to stay on surfaces. These allergens may trigger different allergic conditions for different individuals in the family (or not at all), depending on whether it is the airway or the skin that is sensitised to the allergen.

Role of house dust mites in AD

There is some evidence that house dust mites can trigger AD lesions:

1. After bronchial provocation testing studies with house dust mites, AD lesions may occur. This was shown in a number of well-controlled studies in the lung function lab.
2. In other studies it was shown that AD improved by cleaning the patients' bedrooms, especially in children (results were not convincing in adults).
3. In the blood of patients with AD, specific lymphocytes were detected that start proliferating after contact with house dust mites, suggesting that house dust mites are able to induce inflammation in these patients.
4. When house dust mites are applied on the skin of AD patients by patch testing, new AD lesions can be induced. These skin reactions, which are delayed in time (positive after 24–72 hours), did not occur in allergic asthma and allergic rhinitis, and, therefore, are specific for AD. Microscopy of the patch test reactions shows many similarities to the clinically involved skin in AD.

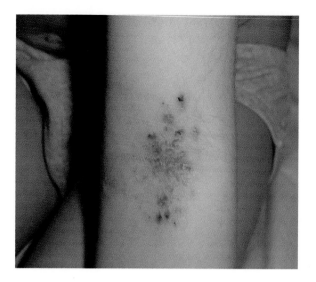

Fig. 4.2 Eczema triggered by house dust mites.

These different types of evidence suggest involvement of house dust mites in certain patients with AD. Patients with a confirmed allergy to house dust mites should include measures to reduce house dust mite exposure. It is also not possible to aim for zero house dust mite exposure in the home, but instead minimise areas for house dust mites to flourish.

Reducing house dust mites

House dust mites can be reduced by removing their food sources and also by eliminating the dust mites through cleaning, for instances through:

1. Reducing the house dust mites trapped in mattresses, bed sheets, pillows, and pillow cases. Mattresses and pillows should be new and protected with anti-dust-mite covers, and not made with natural materials such as feathers. A thinner mattress will make sunning possible. Bed sheets and pillow cases are to be washed weekly, in water of at least 60°C.
2. Removing areas that trap house dust mites and dead human skin such as carpets, heavy curtains, heavy upholstery, and stuffed toys.

3. Regularly cleaning the home, and with damp cleaning instead of dry dusting.
4. Regularly maintaining the air-conditioning system.
5. Regularly sunning the room.
6. Ensuring that the room is not too humid (not above 55%), which promotes the growth of house dust mites.

Cockroach Particles

Different body parts, droppings and saliva of the cockroach are common inhaled allergens that can trigger allergic conditions, including AD, asthma, and rhinitis. An allergy to cockroach (American and German cockroaches, *Periplaneta Americana* and *Blatella germanica* respectively) is mostly associated with a severe house dust mite allergy, and is able to trigger asthma attacks. Cockroaches thrive in (i) warm hiding places, (ii) moist areas, and (iii) with food sources such as food (from trash and scraps), starch, newspapers, book-binding materials, and wallpaper pastes. The allergen particle sizes of cockroaches tend to be large and settle on surfaces. They not only can trigger allergic conditions, but also carry bacteria.

Reducing cockroaches

To minimise cockroach growth, their food source, water and places that can be their shelter should be removed.

1. Remove their food source by storing food in containers and not leaving food exposed, including pet food. Crumbs and spilled drinks should be cleaned and dishes washed. Areas such as stoves and the dining table are also prone to have fallen food.
2. Sweep and mop the floor and reduce clutter in the home.
3. Leaky pipes and drainage areas are possible shelters for cockroaches; fix any leaky drainage.
4. Plug holes and cracks to prevent cockroaches crawling in from outside of the home.
5. Cockroach baits can be used.

Pet Allergens

Cat and dog allergens are the third common inhaled allergens in Asia and can trigger allergic conditions, including AD, asthma, and rhinitis. The allergen in cat dander is a glycoprotein, Fel d1, that is secreted by the cat's sebaceous glands and found in the cat's skin and saliva. The allergen in dog dander is Can f 1, that is found in the dog's saliva and dander. A person who is constantly in contact with the pet may not realise they have an allergy due to chronic daily exposure to the pet, inducing a constant state of hyper-sensitivity of the airways or skin.

For those with a confirmed pet allergy, removing the pet will improve the allergic condition. Washing the pet outside of the home and keeping the pet outside of the bedroom may not sufficiently remove pet allergen to result in an improvement of the AD. It is also possible to have pet dander in the homes of those who do not own pets, as pet dander can catch onto clothes and be brought home. The allergen particle sizes of cat dander tend to be light and airborne, while those of dog dander tend to be heavier and stays on surface.

Reducing pet dander

For those who have a cat or dog allergy, but do not own pets, avoid long visits to homes with pets. Medication can be taken before the visit, or wearing long sleeves and pants can help. For those who keep pets, measures can be taken to reduce contact with the pet dander such as:

1. Keeping the pet outdoors and out of the bedroom and car.
2. Clean furniture, walls, floors, and wooden surfaces.
3. Avoid clutter and surfaces such as carpet and upholstered furniture that trap the pet dander.
4. Clean the bedding weekly.
5. Wear a mask when vacuuming and also wet wipe or mop the house, instead of dry dusting that stirs the allergen into the air.
6. Use an air cleaner for at least four hours per day.
7. Clean and wash the pet regularly, and do so outside of the home.
8. Wash hands, shower and change clothes after contact with the pet.

Pollen

Pollen is a group of microscopic grains needed for plant reproduction, and the common types of pollen that induce allergic reactions are those of plain-looking trees, grasses and weeds whose pollen are small, light and dry and transported by wind. During a pollen season, the pollen concentration in the air is high and can trigger allergic reactions and conditions, including asthma, seasonal rhinitis (hay fever), eczema, and hives. For tropical countries, like Singapore, pollen allergy is very uncommon. The common plants whose pollen trigger allergic reactions are ragweed, sagebrush, redroot pigweed, lamb's quarter, Russian thistle, and English plantain. The common grass that produce highly allergenic pollen are Timothy grass, Kentucky bluegrass, Bermuda grass, Johnson grass, redtop grass, orchard grass, rye grass, and sweet vernal grass. The most common allergenic tree pollen are birch oak, beech, ash, aspen, cottonwood, elm, mulberry, willow, hickory, pecan, box elder, and cedar.

For those with a pollen allergy, it is not sufficient to stay away from the source of pollen, i.e the tree, plant or weed. This is because the pollen is airborne and can be carried from a far distance. Instead, it is better to be aware of pollen count, which is usually higher in the afternoon for most pollens (different for varying pollen types), higher on hot, dry and windy days, and lower when it is cold and wet. Keep windows closed, at home and in the car, and use air-conditioning during the pollen seasons. Dry clothes and bedding inside the home or use a dryer. Change clothing and shower after coming home from the outdoors.

Contact Allergens

Contact allergens are substances that are recognised by the allergic person's immune system as being harmful. After a sensitisation process, whereby the first time the skin comes into contact with the allergen, the immune system recognises it as a foreign harmful particle through a type IV immune response or delayed type immune response, a subsequent exposure, even to a small amount, will induce inflammation of the skin. Patients with AD are susceptible to allergic contact dermatitis due to their damaged skin barrier.

This is more common in adults than in children and is distinguished from irritant contact dermatitis, whereby the immune system is not involved.

The common contact allergens are:

Plants

Plants such as poison ivy, poison oak, poison sumac and cashew (*Anacardeaceae* family) contain urushiol oil that is highly allergenic. Other plants that commonly trigger allergic skin reactions are aster, daisy, sunflower, Rhus trees, daffodils, tulips, chrysanthemums, and primula. When a person's limbs come into contact with the plant and an allergic reaction is triggered, the rash is usually linear with crisscrossing lines resembling the contact points. Other parts of the skin can also develop a rash if the sticky sap of the plant is transferred, for instance to the face or body. A rash can also be triggered by fruit peels, such as mango peel.

Hair dyes and straighteners

Hair dye and straightener products contain many chemicals that can trigger both irritant contact dermatitis and allergic contact dermatitis. The chemical that commonly triggers allergic reactions is paraphenylenediamine (PPD), which can trigger mild to severe reactions in different individuals. The allergic reaction may occur on the face, eyelids, ears, and neck. It is also possible to be cross-reactive to other chemicals such as azo dyes, benzocaine, and para-amino benzoic acid. Other chemicals in hair dye products that can trigger rashes are cobalt and glyceryl thioglycolate. It is best to avoid hair dye once there is an allergy.

Nickel

Nickel is present in earrings, jewellery, studs, zippers, belt buckles, watch straps, clothing fasteners, coins, keys, mobile phones, and eyeglass frames. The allergic reaction occurs on the parts of skin in contact with nickel. It is also possible to have cross-reactivity to other metals, such as cobalt and palladium. For patients with nickel allergy, it is best to avoid body piercing and avoid wearing jewellery, accessories or clothing with nickel. Choose instead alternative material such as stainless steel, pure sterling silver, platinum, at least 14-karat gold, and plastic-coated accessories.

Latex (natural rubber)

Latex can cause allergic reactions, particularly for those whose occupation include wearing rubber gloves or work in rubber-related manufacturing. There is also latex allergy observed in those with repeated spine or urinary tract surgeries, and in children with spina bifida. In Singapore, almost 50% of children with spina bifida suffer from latex allergy. Exposure to latex is not limited to contact, but can also be via mucous membranes, inhalation, and blood. The allergic reactions can occur immediately or be delayed, and be as severe as anaphylaxis. There is cross-reactivity between latex and certain food proteins, such as those of banana, avocado, chestnut, kiwi, apricot, papaya, and tomato.

If there is a latex allergy, latex products are to be avoided including those labelled as *safe latex*. Products that contain latex include balloons, rubber bands, shoe soles, pacifiers, and condoms. Alternatives to latex (natural rubber) are synthetic rubber such as neoprene, nitrile, butyl or petroleum-based synthetic polymers.

Bacterial Colonisation of Skin

Bacterial colonisation, particularly with *Staphylococcus aureus*, is very common in patients with AD and found in so-called normal skin and in eczematous skin lesions. There are studies that have correlated the severity of AD with *S. aureus* colonisation. The *S. aureus* bacteria produces toxins that are able to act as superantigens that activate inflammatory cells (T lymphocytes), resulting in skin inflammation. Moreover, *S. aureus* is able to induce IgE production in the skin. *S. aureus* bacteria can also cause skin infections, such as impetigo. Moreover, for patients with AD who scratch their skin and cause skin damage, the warm, moist and broken skin barrier make it an ideal environment for bacterial colonisation.

Taken together, *Staphylococcus aureus* colonisation of the skin can maintain skin inflammation through the following mechanisms:

1. Production of toxins (proteases) that damage the skin.
2. Production of superantigens, inducing inflammation.
3. Production of specific-IgE, inducing IgE-mediated inflammation.

For patients with eczema, it is important to take measures to reduce the amount of *S. aureus* bacteria. This can be achieved by following good hygiene practices, and:

1. Treating the eczema so that there is less itch and less scratching.
2. Cleaning the eczema lesions with diluted chlorhexidine gluconate or other non-irritating antiseptics, such as potassium permanganate or zinc–copper sulphate.
3. For children, bleach bath can be prepared twice a week for soaking of 5 to 10 minutes.
4. The best way to keep bacteria low on the skin is regular swimming (three to four times per week) in chlorinated water (swimming pool) and to catch the swimming pool water with a moisturiser (no shower after swimming). For those who are sensitive to chlorine, a quick rinse can be taken followed by moisturisation immediately after. Moreover, swimming is healthy for the lungs and at the same time the child stays outdoors (no contact with house dust mites). However, direct contact with the sun should be avoided, particularly for those with active eczema lesions.

Should symptoms of bacterial infection be observed, such as painful, tender skin, fever or the development of pus, blister or boils, sore and protruding lymph nodes, a doctor ought to be consulted and topical antibiotic cream or oral antibiotics may be prescribed. However, antibiotics should **be avoided as much as possible**, as long-term usage can induce bacterial resistance. If there is fever, chills accompanied by low blood pressure, fainting, muscle aches, emergency treatment should be sought as sepsis- or toxic shock syndrome might have occurred.

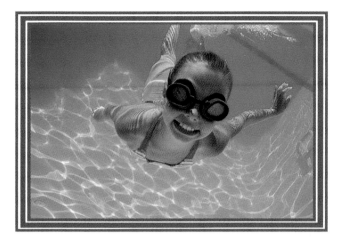

Fig. 4.3   Swimming can aid in keeping bacteria count low.

A note on methicillin-resistant S. aureus bacteria (MRSA)

Due to the rise of MRSA (bacteria resistant to common antibiotics methicillin) and also increasing resistance to cloxacillin and erythromycin, prevention of bacterial colonisation and consequent infection should be the focus of eczema management. Regular swimming seems the best!

Stress

Stress can trigger flare-ups of AD or worsen it through various possible mechanisms: (i) stress impairs skin barrier function allowing more irritants and allergens to penetrate, and induces higher moisture loss, via inflammatory reactions (i.e. increase of nerve growth factors and increase in cytokine production); (ii) stress lowers the ability of the body's immune system to defend against infection. Apart from stress resulting in increased skin inflammation, stress can also induce stress behaviour, such as scratching or rubbing of skin, resulting in further skin damage.

To avoid stress triggering or worsening eczema, older children and adults should adopt stress relaxation techniques and lifestyle options such as sufficient sleep, breathing or exercises that are relaxing and seeking support through a local group. AD itself is a stressful condition that commonly leads to disrupted sleep and higher stress, and thus an active positive attitude ought to be adopted to manage the condition.

Infections

Fever and respiratory infections, such as influenza (flu) can trigger AD flare-ups, particularly in children. The higher temperature itself triggers eczema (through an increased metabolism, thereby increasing inflammation). Moreover, certain viruses may partially paralyse the immune system, allowing allergic inflammation to become more intense. A more vigilant skincare regime should be applied during the fever or flu to ensure that the skin inflammation remains suppressed.

Hormonal Changes

Eczema flare-ups are observed in some patients during periods of hormonal changes, such as during pregnancy, puberty, premenstrual and post-menopause. Certain hormones reduce the skin thickness or predispose the immune system to allergic reactions, and their impact varies between gender and age. Adopting a skincare regime and healthy lifestyle can assist to protect the skin barrier.

Irritant Substances

Irritant substances can trigger hypersensitive reactions (increase inflammation directly) by penetrating the skin barrier, activating different inflammatory cells. Sometimes, it is difficult to differentiate between allergic contact dermatitis and irritant contact dermatitis, as its symptoms are similar. In general, irritant substances can trigger allergic contact dermatitis by activating an antigen–antibody reaction, while in irritant dermatitis this does not occur.

Broadly speaking, irritant substances are classified into those that (i) trigger a primary irritation, and (ii) trigger an allergic reaction after sensitisation. Strong chemicals typically trigger a primary irritation, such as hydrochloric acid in fertilisers and paints, and sodium hydroxide in detergents, disinfectants and cleaning products. Protective gear such as gloves and long sleeve clothing can help to reduce contact with these chemicals. Moisturisers are studied to have a protective effect against irritant substances, as it forms another layer above the skin barrier.

Other ingredients in skincare products, such as fragrance, lanolin, propylene glycol, preservatives (parabens, benzyl alcohol, formaldehyde releasers), sodium lauryl sulphate, triclosan and natural ingredients such as vitamin E, pantothenol, aloe vera, and chamomile can also trigger inflammatory skin reactions. Patch testing can be used to diagnose contact dermatitis. This is mainly used in adults with AD. Once a substance is confirmed to trigger a hypersensitive reaction, avoiding the substance can help to reduce instances of eczema flare-ups.

Other substances such as soaps with a high pH level and hot water can dry the skin and remove its natural oil, making the skin more porous for irritants and allergens. As the skin barrier of eczema skin is impaired, hot water should be avoided, as this will further exacerbate moisture loss from the skin.

Perspiration has been found to irritate skin, especially in children with active eczema lesions. Certain wool with scratchy fibres, or processed with chemicals, also can irritate the skin. Moreover, thicker wool material can trap heat, which is a trigger for eczema for some. Cotton clothing is recommended.

Heat

Heat can be a trigger of eczema flare-ups for some, while for others extreme changes in temperature can trigger flare-up. This is through non-specific triggering of inflammatory reactions of the skin. In patients whose eczema is triggered by heat, air-conditioning can be helpful.

Cold Climate

Cold climate during winter season is characterised by dry and cold air, with low humidity that can strip moisture from the skin. The forced heating system indoors also reduces humidity or may contain circulating inhaled allergens. A thicker moisturiser can be applied for longer lasting effect and protection during the winter months.

Pollutant

Air pollutants and cigarette smoke may also irritate the skin. It is best to stay indoors, or to wear long sleeves and apply moisturiser before heading outdoors.

Mechanical Irritation

Rubbing of the skin due to itch can set off the itch-scratch vicious cycle where the itch leads to scratching, which causes further inflammation due to the vulnerability of the damaged skin. Parents can assist to distract their child from scratching by positive reinforcement of not scratching and alternative activities. Keeping the bacteria low on the skin will reduce itch, as it has been shown that itch can be maintained by bacterial colonisation. Keeping fingernails short and smooth reduces damage done by scratching.

Alcohol

Alcohol has resulted in eczema flare-ups in some adults, although the underlying mechanisms are not fully known. Allergy to alcohol is uncommon, although other ingredients in the wine can trigger hypersensitive reactions.

Mom Asks, Doc Answers!

MarcieMom: *Is it possible for a fetus to be sensitised or does sensitisation start from birth?*

Professor Hugo: Studies on prenatal sensitisation are difficult to perform, mainly for ethical reasons. However, from the observational studies (there are no intervention studies), it seems that allergen exposure of the pregnant woman (food and inhalants), also called prenatal exposure, has little influence on the foetus. In contrast, it was shown that foetal lymphocytes become active from week 20 of pregnancy. It seems, however, that the placenta acts as a huge filter for allergens. Therefore, we accept that sensitisation mainly occurs after birth, although more studies on the subject are needed, and prenatal sensitisation might exist.

MarcieMom: *Does a certain category of allergen, say food allergen, take a shorter or longer time to be sensitised to as opposed to inhaled or contact allergens?*

Professor Hugo: Yes. During the first year of life, allergies are mainly against food. The most common food allergies in infants are; cow's milk (number one), egg, soy, and wheat. Egg allergy is the most common allergy in babies with eczema. In contrast, allergic sensitisation against inhalants (such as house dust mites) takes longer, usually two to three years, and is extremely rare during the first year of life.

MarcieMom: *Will the severity of allergic reactions alter for a particular allergen? For instance, is it possible for a baby to have a mild reaction and subsequently, the reaction turns more severe with increased exposure?*

Professor Hugo: Yes, this is possible. Once an allergy has occurred it is better to avoid the allergen. Repeated exposure can induce more severe allergy.

MarcieMom: *Has it been studied whether it is the food allergy that results in severe atopic dermatitis or is it a severe atopic dermatitis that leads to food allergy?*

Professor Hugo: Both! The relation between food allergy and eczema is very complex. Many possibilities exist. Eczema can induce food allergy, and food allergy can make eczema worse. It is also possible that both are present in a child without influencing each other.

MarcieMom: *Could food allergens seem to be less common as a trigger for older children because other triggers mask its presentation?*

Professor Hugo: No, studies using objective tools such as provocation testing have shown that food allergy is more common in young children, especially in infants with severe eczema.

MarcieMom: *Is there any association between the severity of food allergy to the severity of atopic dermatitis in children?*

Professor Hugo: Not really. A severe food allergy can occur without eczema worsening, and manifest itself as urticaria or anaphylaxis, while a mild food allergy can maintain eczema. However, usually more allergic reactions to food and inhalants can be found in severe eczema. Severe eczema can also exist without food allergy. Many variations are possible.

MarcieMom: *There seem to be more parents who view their children as having food allergies than having eczema, though a skin rash is a reaction from the food allergy. How do doctors "categorise" patients if they have both?*

Professor Hugo: Food allergy and eczema can exist separately, but can also be present in one child. Usually, children with eczema and with food allergy are categorised as: atopic eczema with an underlying food allergy. But one should remember that the most common manifestation of food allergy is urticaria, not eczema.

MarcieMom: *Is exercise-induced allergy common in children, and if so, which are the common foods consumed before the exercise that triggers such an allergic reaction?*

Professor Hugo: It is not common, but it seems to be increasing. Recently we see more wheat-induced exercise-induced allergy. This is also seen in Thailand and in Japan. Other foods that can induce exercise-induced allergy are seafood.

MarcieMom: *Which are the common cross-reactivities in children?*

Professor Hugo: In Singapore we see cross-reactivity between house dust mites and seafood (due to tropomyosin). In Europe and USA, the most common cross-reactivity is between pollen and fruits/vegetables.

MarcieMom: *How can one distinguish food allergy from food sensitivity?*

Professor Hugo: Food allergy is caused by an immunological reaction, usually IgE-mediated, and does occur after ingestion of small amounts. Food sensitivity or better hypersensitivity is usually not immunological, and occurs mainly after large amounts. It occurs because the body doesn't accept the food. Many causes exist, such as lactase deficiency. Also, infected food (food poisoning) is a type of food hypersensitivity.

MarcieMom: *What are the common conditions related to consumption of shrimps? What are the symptoms of shrimp allergy?*

Professor Hugo: Shrimp allergy is the most common food allergy in older children in Singapore. Usually it manifests not differently from other food allergies. Symptoms are urticaria and angioedema (swelling of lips, eyes). In severe cases anaphylaxis occurs (affecting airways or intestines), which might lead to anaphylactic shock.

MarcieMom: *There has been a lot more focus lately on gluten-free diet. I've read that wheat allergen tends to provoke a higher number of IgE antibodies in patients with atopic dermatitis, thus removing gluten for these AD patients with gluten sensitivity can alleviate the eczema symptoms. Is that right? What is the study in this area, especially for children who are growing and need a balanced diet?*

Professor Hugo: Gluten intolerance is a different problem, manifesting as coeliac disease. Eczema and coeliac disease have a different underlying mechanism. A lot has been written on its involvement in eczema, but not really on a scientific base. Wheat allergy is uncommon in eczema. Most children with eczema have no problems with gluten. The literature is absolutely not convincing.

MarcieMom: *On the elimination diet, is it acceptable for parents to conduct this on their own to try to figure out which foods are triggering the eczema flare-ups? For how long should such a diet be carried out, and how many foods should be excluded at the start?*

Professor Hugo: My answer is: Don't do it yourself as it can be dangerous for the child. An elimination diet is hardly necessary in eczema. If indicated, it should be designed by a doctor or dietician who is specialised in eczema. In my own practice I almost never use it. The better method is to identify the food to which the child is allergic and to eliminate it from the diet.

MarcieMom: *If food packaging has labels using words such as "may contain" a certain potential food allergen, should those with confirmed food allergy read it as the packaged food has the allergen and not consume it?*

Professor Hugo: Don't take any risk. "May contain" foods should also be avoided, as even small amounts of food can induce an allergic reaction.

MarcieMom: *When should someone suspect he/she has a house dust mite allergy? This is particularly so if the person has been living in the same home and symptoms of house dust mite allergy come and go?*

Professor Hugo: A house dust mite allergy is mostly impossible to diagnose through history, as there are few specific symptoms. Only sneezing in the morning is a specific symptom, but is not present in all patients with house dust mite allergy. The diagnosis is based on a positive allergy test (skin prick test or specific IgE in the blood).

MarcieMom: *In the support group sharing sessions that I facilitate, a few mothers shared about the large amount of skin their children shed from a night's sleep. Do you recommend that additional effort be made to remove dead skin for those with a house dust mite allergy? How often should the beddings be changed and the room be cleaned?*

Professor Hugo: This has never been studied. However, it seems logical as dead skin is the preferred food of house dust mites. Usually we recommend looking at the condition of the child in the first place. More rigorous measures are advised if the eczema persists.

MarcieMom: *Are there hypoallergenic cats and dogs or is it a myth?*

Professor Hugo: A myth, as the saliva of pets also contains allergens.

MarcieMom: *Does living with a cat help to prevent a cat allergy? And is this studied to be the same versus living with a dog to prevent a dog allergy from young?*

Professor Hugo: Be careful with this statement, as we don't have intervention studies, only observations (and allergic families tend to keep fewer pets). However, from the observational studies it seems that keeping a pet (cat or dog) early in life is protective for allergy, probably because of the increased bacterial load to the immune system caused by pets. Once you have an allergy to a pet, removal is still the best advice.

MarcieMom: *Studies on whether the same allergy can be passed on to children seem to be contradicting. In your view, can a child acquire the same pet allergy as the parent? And will this allergy manifest in the same manner?*

Professor Hugo: The potential to develop allergy is genetically determined, nothing more. Children can develop different allergies compared to their parents. This is dependent on environmental contact with allergens.

MarcieMom: *I often see in forums where the grandparents have a pet and the parents suspect their child have an allergy to the pet. Does it make a difference to the development of a pet allergy whether (a) the pet is at home, (b) the pet is at the grandparents' home and the child visits the home regularly, or (c) the pet is at the grandparents' home and the grandparents visit the child regularly?*

Professor Hugo: This has never been studied, but any contact with pets can induce allergy. The more contact the higher the risk. However, cat allergen is a very airborne allergen (very light) and is impossible to avoid, similar to house dust mites. This is not the case for dog allergen.

MarcieMom: *Pollen is light and can be stirred into the air easily. Does having an air cleaner help with removing pollen and is there certain feature of the air cleaner to look out for to ensure it cleans the air more than it stirs the pollen into the air?*

Professor Hugo: During the pollen season it is impossible to avoid pollen, especially outdoors. Air cleaner studies on this have not been performed — at least, there have been no clinical studies. However, in Singapore we don't have a pollen season and no pollen allergies.

MarcieMom: *Which fruits tend to trigger allergic reactions from touching the peel? Will slicing more of the flesh nearer to the peel help to reduce the possibility of triggering a reaction?*

Professor Hugo: In theory all fruits can induce allergy, but fruit allergy is uncommon, even in children with eczema, except peanut and nut allergy. Details of your question have not been studied.

MarcieMom: *Do the pesticides found on vegetables and fruits also trigger allergic reactions?*

Professor Hugo: This is unknown from studies. However, pesticides are not proteins and therefore are unlikely to induce allergic reactions.

MarcieMom: *I read that paraphenylenediamine (PPD) is banned in certain European countries due to the allergic reactions it can trigger, including anaphylaxis. Is there a way for someone to know if he/she has a severe reaction to PPD before getting the hair dye?*

Professor Hugo: In children PPD is not a common problem, and there are no diagnostic tests to predict a reaction. PPD is mainly a problem in adult hairdressers causing contact dermatitis. This can be diagnosed by a patch test.

MarcieMom: *How long does it usually take for a health care worker to develop a latex allergy? Is it possible to know before taking on that occupation?*

Professor Hugo: Prediction of latex allergy is impossible, and the time to develop sensitisation varies strongly. In children, latex allergy is mainly a problem in spina bifida patients.

MarcieMom: *Are there babies who are more genetically predisposed to bacterial colonisation? Or will atopic dermatitis always precede bacterial colonisation?*

Professor Hugo: We all are colonised with bacteria; this is an absolute necessity to maintain a good skin barrier function. However, children with congenital skin barrier defects, such as filaggrin deficiency, seem to have an altered bacterial colonisation (including less diversity of bacteria on the skin), which might induce skin inflammation and the onset of eczema. More studies on the subject are necessary, as this is a relatively new finding.

MarcieMom: *Previously we mentioned about eczema patches "migrating" from certain parts of the skin to another. Does this have anything to do with S. aureus colonisation moving from one part of the skin to another?*

Professor Hugo: Probably not, but we don't know the underlying mechanism of the migration of eczema lesions.

MarcieMom: *What is the treatment for those with recurring bacterial colonisation and infection?*

Professor Hugo: Almost all children with eczema have abnormal skin colonisation with *Staphylococcus aureus*. Regular swimming is the best approach. Cleaning the skin with a mild antiseptic is also advisable. Antibiotics should be avoided, as they induce bacterial resistance.

MarcieMom: *Where apart from skin are common places where S. aureus bacteria reside?*

Professor Hugo: Mainly in the nose. Keeping the nose clean is advisable. Sometimes we treat with a short course of antibiotics, because antiseptics can cause irritation of the nose. Nasal antibiotics are only used if really necessary (i.e. persistent skin infections) and always as a short course.

MarcieMom: *I noticed that my child had noticeably more itchy and "rashy" skin when ill and I now tend to lower her temperature more aggressively, via medication and patting with a cold towel. Is that necessary?*

Professor Hugo: Fever will stimulate metabolism, including inflammatory reactions. Keeping fever under control is advisable.

MarcieMom: *Is eczema triggered during hormonal changes long-lasting or will the eczema disappear after the period of hormonal change?*

Professor Hugo: Usually these flare-ups are temporarily, but exceptions do exist.

MarcieMom: *What is the ingredient in soap that can irritate the skin? There are many products marketed at being the same pH level as the skin. Does pH level play a role in whether there is a hypersensitive reaction?*

Professor Hugo: Use soaps without fragrance or perfume and with a neutral ph. However, what you use during bathing is less important than what you use after bathing: *moisturising* after bathing is the most important action. However, there are no good clinical studies on which soap to use. Therefore, usually I recommend using soap and a moisturiser that the child likes. Small molecules in soap (preservatives, fragrances) may induce contact eczema.

MarcieMom: *Will sweat that has dried off the skin still irritate the skin? Similarly for clothes soaked in sweat, should additional measures be taken to wash them (i.e. any sweat residue that irritates?)*

Professor Hugo: Sweat and saliva can irritate the skin. Never moisturise on a sweaty skin, but have a short shower first. Clothes should be washed and rinsed without specific precautions.

MarcieMom: *Is there any preventive measure that one can take before relocating to a country with a different climate?*

Professor Hugo: Be sure that you know the underlying mechanisms of your child's eczema, especially all the triggers. Avoidance, wherever you are, is the rule.

MarcieMom: *It is commonly heard that eczema worsens or improves during a holiday. Is there any way that a person can accurately guess which is the trigger or triggers that make the difference in his/her skin?*

Professor Hugo: We attribute this to the different environment (different allergens) and to less stress. But there are no good studies on this.

MarcieMom: *How about negligence to dutifully follow the skin care routine during travelling? Do you see it in your practice?*

Professor Hugo: It happens, and it is important to emphasise to parents their responsibility.

CHAPTER 5

Eczema Prevention

In the previous chapter, triggers of eczema were discussed and it was emphasised that avoiding known triggers helps in controlling eczema. However, as eczema is a condition that significantly lowers the quality of life of children and adults, the question parents frequently ask is whether there is a way to prevent its onset altogether (also known as primary prevention). Till now, despite many studies on primary prevention, it seems impossible to prevent eczema completely. This is mainly due to (i) a strong genetic predisposition, and (ii) the multi-factorial conditioning of eczema, involving a wide spectrum of triggering factors. There are, however, certain areas in primary prevention that have been more extensively studied. These areas will be discussed in further detail in this chapter.

Breastfeeding

Breast milk is the best milk for babies, and it is very likely that no formula milk will ever be better. Breastfeeding is recommended by the World Health Organisation, and the current guideline is to exclusively breastfeed till the infant is six month old, and to continue providing the child with breast milk (complemented by foods) till up to two years old. Breast milk is recognised as a well-balanced nutrition for the baby's growth and colostrum; the breast milk produced during pregnancy contains antibodies and immunoglobulines that strengthen the immunity of the newborn.

The role of breastfeeding in primary prevention is generally accepted, although good scientific studies on breastfeeding are difficult to perform and are generally lacking. It is accepted that exclusive breastfeeding for up to the age of four months is able to reduce the risk for eczema and also has a protective effect on allergic diseases. There are also studies indicating that exclusive breastfeeding till the age of three months reduces atopic dermatitis for children with a family history of atopy.

However, in other studies the role of breastfeeding was found to be less pronounced, and even contradicting conclusions were published, suggesting breastfeeding can be harmful. Reasons for this can be found in the methodology of the studies, and in the fact that it is impossible to study breastfeeding using a double-blind, placebo-controlled study design. An example of this is the fact that mothers of allergic families are more keen to breast feed, resulting in the false positive notion that allergy is linked (a consequence) of breastfeeding.

Despite contradicting studies on the protective effect of prolonged breastfeeding on eczema, it should be noted that breast milk has remained the most well-balanced and appropriate nutrition for a baby. Breast milk has been studied to provide protective effects over other diseases and long-term health benefits, including over gastrointestinal infections, type II diabetes, obesity, blood pressure, and cholesterol. Moreover, no study was ever published in which it was shown that any other milk is better than breast milk. Therefore, the logical conclusion is that breastfeeding is the best feeding procedure in the primary prevention of eczema and other allergic diseases. However, breastfeeding cannot prevent all allergies. Studies on the improvement of anti-allergic features of breast milk (i.e. certain cytokines, such as IL-10, in breast milk have an inhibiting effect on allergy development) are underway, and it is very likely that breast milk will always be the best milk for preventing allergy and eczema.

Therefore:

> "No milk is better than breast milk in primary prevention of eczema and allergy."

Role of Pregnancy and the Lactation Diet

Pregnancy Diet

There are a number of studies on the role of diets during pregnancy on the development of eczema in the offspring. These studies showed that any diet during pregnancy has no effect on eczema in the offspring. More recent studies, however, have suggested that extra vitamin D or poly-unsaturated fatty acids (fish oil) might have some protective effect.

In the "Management of Food Allergy" Clinical Practice Guidelines 2/2010 by Academy of Medicine Singapore and Ministry of Health Singapore, there is also no recommendation on avoidance of foods during pregnancy due to a lack of conclusive studies.

Lactation Diet

One of the most notable guidelines comes from The American Academy of Pediatrics (AAP) in 2008, stating: "… *there is a lack of convincing evidence for a long-term protective effect of maternal diet during lactation on atopic disease in childhood.*"

The foods that a mother eats can be transmitted into her breast milk. For instance, antigens of cow's milk, chicken egg and peanuts can be detected in breast milk for up to hours after consuming the foods. Therefore, in some children with food allergy as a cause of their eczema, avoidance of these foods by the mother might be advised. However, there is no strong scientific evidence on this type of intervention, and it is still inconclusive whether avoidance of these foods is able to prevent or delay the onset of eczema.

With regard to which foods can prevent childhood eczema if consumed during pregnancy and nursing, there is no conclusive study although certain studies point to intake of omega-3 supplements for mothers with eczema can reduce eczema in the baby during pregnancy and nursing. With regard to antioxidants, there is no strong association between its consumption during pregnancy and childhood eczema.

Therefore:

1. A diet during pregnancy has no effect upon the development of eczema in the offspring. A well-balanced diet is essential for the pregnant and lactating mother, but one should check with the gynecologist on supplements such as omega-3, folic acid, iron, and multi-vitamins.

2. Breast milk is the appropriate nutrition for an infant, and its nutritional value does depend on the diet and lifestyle of the mother. Alcohol, nicotine and caffeine should be avoided or reduced as these can be transmitted to both the fetus and the baby via breast milk. Alcohol consumption had been associated with higher IgE levels and overconsumption presents a risk of toxicity. Tobacco smoke has been linked with an increase in Th2 cytokines, specific IgE levels and higher incidences of bronchitis asthma.

Role of Hypoallergenic Milk

Hypoallergenic milk refers to partially and extensively hydrolysed formula, where the protein in cow's milk formula has been hydrolysed or broken down into smaller protein chains that are less likely to trigger allergic reactions. Hydrolysed milk should not be taken as a replacement for breast milk.

Various Types of Hypoallergenic Formula

CLASS	CARBOHYDRATE SOURCE	PROTEIN SOURCE	AVAILABILITY
Partially hydrolysed formula	Corn, sucrose or lactose	Partially hydrolysed cow's milk protein	In supermarkets
Extensively hydrolysed formula	Corn or sucrose	Extensively hydrolysed cow's milk protein	By prescription
Free amino acid-based	Corn or sucrose	Amino acids	By prescription

The fact is that eczema and cow's milk allergy are different diseases, and cow's milk allergy is involved only in a minority of children with eczema. However, it has been shown in a few studies that hydrolysed formulas (extensively and partially) can prevent the development of eczema. The problem is that eczema cannot be predicted. Therefore, it is impossible to select the newborn at risk for eczema. Moreover, studies on the protective effect of hydrolysed formulas on eczema are still not conclusive, and there is no study that compares hydrolysed formula versus breast milk in offering long-term protective benefits for eczema. For high-risk infants who could not be 100% breastfed, there is limited evidence to support the use of hydrolysed formulas. Compared to cow's milk, there are a few studies that reported lower incidence of atopic dermatitis for high-risk children being fed hydrolysed or partially hydrolysed formula, including a preventive effect up to the age of 10 years. There is no conclusive evidence to support giving the child a hypoallergenic formula after weaning to protect him from allergic diseases.

A note on switching formulas

Breast milk is the recommended nutrition for an infant; it not only provides the essential nutrients required, but can also cater to the infant's varying nutrition needs. There are protective effects in breast milk that cannot be replicated in formula milk. Breast milk is the only "living milk" containing immune cells and immune mediators. If formula milk has to be used, cow's milk remains the first alternative to breast milk due to the similarities in whey and casein proteins. Some parents switch their infants to other forms of milk, due to colic or rashes. The decision to switch formula types should not be taken without consulting a physician. Each alternative, including cow's milk, has downsides that breast milk does not have, and is always less suitable for babies.

Hydrolysed formula is bitter and has sweeteners added to make it palatable, along with lactose alternatives such as corn syrup and modified corn starch that are artificial sugars.

Goat's milk has similar protein chains as cow's milk and therefore is not recommended as an alternative for a child with cow's milk allergy. Soy formula is not recommended for infants who also have an allergy to soy (and infants with cow's milk allergy have a higher likelihood of soy allergy). By itself, soy milk lacks various important amino acids and calcium, and therefore, soy formula has added nutrients to ensure suitability for various age groups.

A note on starting solids

It is recommended to start solids at six months of age. There is no evidence to support the delayed introduction of solids beyond six months to prevent eczema.

Studies are not convincing for the recommendation of delayed introduction of eggs, peanuts and fish. However, as egg allergy is the most common food allergy in eczema, many physicians advise not to give eggs during the first year of life. Delaying an introduction of certain foods may delay exposure to the potential food allergen till the child's immunity is more developed, but it has also been postulated to deprive the window for a developing immunity to accept and tolerate the foods.

Role of Bacterial Products

Bacterial products have been studied for use in eczema prevention and treatment. Part of the interest in bacterial products come from the earlier mentioned Hygiene Hypothesis, where a decreased bacterial load resulted in less simulation of the immune system, such as less developed Th2 features. Moreover, a decreased diversity of skin microbiota and abnormalities in gut flora has been reported in children with allergy and with eczema. Therefore, it was postulated that increasing the bacterial load early in life may suppress the development of allergic conditions.

Probiotics are defined as "live micro-organisms, which when consumed in adequate amounts confer a health effect on the host." The International Scientific Association for Probiotics and Prebiotics issued a clarification in 2009 that probiotics used in foods should be (i) alive when administered and (ii) have undergone controlled evaluation to document health benefits in the target host. Prebiotics, on the other hand, are "non-digestible sugars that beneficially affect the host by selectively stimulating the growth and/or activity of one or a limited number of bacterial species already established in the colon, and thus in effect improve host health." Synbiotics are defined as "mixtures of probiotics and prebiotics that beneficially affect the host by improving the survival and implantation of live microbial dietary supplements in the gastrointestinal tract of the host."

With regard to eczema prevention, studies noted a decrease in incidence of eczema in breastfed infants who had been supplemented by probiotics, taken by the mother, in the last two to eight weeks of pregnancy and up to two years after birth. There were, however, also studies with contradicting results. Formulas containing bacterial products seem to be far less effective.

The type of probiotics vary, though probiotic strains have to be present in billions, and the most commonly studied strains come from the *Lactobacillus* and *Bifidobacteria* groups, such as the *Lactobacillus rhamnosus GG*, *Lactobacillus rhamnosus LC705*, *Bifidobacterium breve Bb99*, *Bifidobacterium animalis ssp. lactis*, *Bifidobacterium bifidum*, *Bifidobacterium lactis and Lactococcus lactis* strains, or a combination of various strains. The protective effect of probiotics for eczema has been seen in certain studies to last till four years old. Probiotics in infant formula mostly did not indicate any protective effect for the onset of eczema, both in studies in Australia and Singapore. Studies on allergy (IgE-mediated reactions) and on respiratory symptoms have failed to show positive results.

With regard to eczema treatment, probiotics have no major role as only a few small studies reported mild improvement of atopic dermatitis after the administration of bacterial products.

More studies on bacterial products are underway, and for the moment it is difficult to conclude on the most effective method of using probiotics as (i) the type and combination of probiotics and its dosage, (ii) duration of administration of bacterial products and when best to do so, (iii) form of administration, (iv) duration of breastfeeding, and (v) interaction with the resident gut flora in the infant and the mother may all play a part in the effectiveness. It is also not conclusive whether the administration of probiotics is more effective for children with a family history of atopy or when the mothers themselves also suffer from allergic disease. Probiotics (of certain strains) supplementation are generally safe for healthy individuals and its benefits are also being studied in many areas, including but not limited to acute diarrhea in children, inflammatory bowel diseases, gastrointestinal infections, and urinary tract infections.

For the moment, it seems that probiotics are mainly effective when taken by the mother, in combination with breastfeeding and started during late pregnancy. Underlying mechanisms seem to be related to an impact on skin and gut flora, indirectly inhibiting the occurrence of eczema, not on IgE-mediated reactions.

Role of Early Moisturising

Allergic sensitisation to inhalants (house dust mite and other) and food can occur through the skin (transdermal), and for babies born with a defective skin barrier, moisturising may prevent transdermal sensitisation. Moisturising also serves to protect against the repeated exposure of irritants. It is also hypothesised that the protection of the skin barrier has an effect on the prevention of the Allergic March. However, studies need to be conducted before early moisturising can be recommended for routine eczema prevention.

Mom Asks, Doc Answers!

MarcieMom: *For mothers who are unable to exclusively breastfeed, what would be your recommendation on the nutrition for the baby?*

Professor Hugo: Most formulas on the market are of good quality, and under extensive control by the authorities. Most babies have no problems with a formula. The problem is that we cannot predict eczema. However, the risk for eczema in the baby is higher in families with eczema. In these babies a partially or extensively hydrolysed formula is recommended, in case breastfeeding is impossible.

MarcieMom: *What ingredients in breast milk provide possible protective effects on childhood eczema which formula milk doesn't have?*

Professor Hugo: This is the subject of intense research, where attempts are made to answer the question: What are the anti-allergic features of breast milk and how can we improve this? From what we know now, it seems that certain cytokines (IL-10, TGF-beta, and others) and certain immunoglobulins, such as IgA, are responsible for suppressing allergy in the baby. The role of prebiotics and probiotics is under study, and little is known on the role of immune cells in breast milk.

MarcieMom: *Are there conclusive studies on the early introduction of food allergens via the mother's diet, either during pregnancy or lactation? Is it more likely to result in a development of allergy or less likely due to earlier exposure?*

Professor Hugo: From the current literature, it seems that any diet of the mother during pregnancy or breastfeeding has little effect on eczema in the baby. However, most studies are observational studies, and there are no good intervention studies.

MarcieMom: *Is it possible that for mothers who have an allergic disease and exclusively breastfeed for longer than four months may actually increase the risk of development of eczema in the child?*

Professor Hugo: There is insufficient data on this. Don't forget that it is very difficult to study breastfeeding. Breast feeding till the age of six months is recommended and the introduction of solids can start at the age of six months. In children with eczema we advise not to give eggs till the age of one, but this is mainly based on experience, not on studies.

MarcieMom: *What is difference between the breast milk of a mother who has allergy and one without? I've read that essential fatty acids may be lower in mothers with allergy?*

Professor Hugo: There are many confounders in this. For the moment there is insufficient data on this. From a few studies from Australia it seems that allergic mothers have less protective cytokines and IgA in their milk, but more studies are needed. The role of fatty acids in eczema has been insufficiently studied.

MarcieMom: *I have come across many mothers who feel guilty when they suspect that their consumption of certain foods (especially during lactation) seems to have triggered an eczema flare-up in the baby. Is it possible, say, for the mother to trigger eczema in the infant after consuming a few prawns or eating a few peanuts? Would that infant have to be genetically predisposed to allergic disease for that to be possible? (I'm asking this so that mothers can gain some clarity and not blame themselves for causing eczema in their children.)*

Professor Hugo: Don't blame yourself if you are breastfeeding. The role of diets in the mother during breastfeeding seems to be very minimal. Of course, a few exceptions exist, and if your baby has an obvious flare-up of eczema after eating a certain food it is better to avoid the food, and talk about it with your physician.

MarcieMom: *Does it make sense to avoid food allergens for an infant who has not exhibited any symptom of food allergy but the father has an allergy to certain foods (not the mother, since she would already be avoiding the foods if a certain food allergy is confirmed)?*

Professor Hugo: That does not make sense, as the prevalence of food allergy is low and as the child can react to other foods, if genetically allergic, according to age.

MarcieMom: *What is your personal recommendation on peanuts? Will you suggest that mothers consider avoiding peanuts, and if so, under what circumstances?*

Professor Hugo: There is contradictory data from the literature, and studies on avoiding peanuts from the UK actually saw an increase of peanut allergy. It is impossible to predict if a child will develop a food allergy, including a peanut allergy, and therefore, I have no specific recommendation. A healthy balanced diet during pregnancy and lactation seems to be more important.

MarcieMom: *What about delaying the introduction of peanuts for high-risk children?*

Professor Hugo: Same answer: It is impossible to predict peanut allergy, and delaying introduction of peanuts is not a guarantee for no peanut allergy.

MarcieMom: *Will you recommend a mother with severe food reaction to modify her pregnancy and lactation diet?*

Professor Hugo: No, I will recommend healthy food.

MarcieMom: *There are also studies on the impact on oral supplements on eczema, taken for an adult. If a food has been studied to improve adult* *eczema, does it also mean it is likely to improve childhood eczema, if taken during pregnancy and nursing?*

Professor Hugo: This has never been shown, and I recommend not to experiment during pregnancy or breastfeeding. After all, the role of supplements in childhood eczema has never been proven.

MarcieMom: *What about alcohol during pregnancy? Is it safe?*

Professor Hugo: Alcohol during pregnancy or breastfeeding should be avoided, as it can have many negative effects on the foetus and baby. The extreme is the so-called "Foetal Alcohol Syndrome." There are some indications that alcohol might act as an epigenetic regulator, inducing eczema, but this needs more study.

MarcieMom: *Is extensively hydrolysed milk formula commonly prescribed, and why?*

Professor Hugo: It is commonly prescribed, mainly because we cannot predict cow's milk allergy, and most physicians don't want to take the risk. There is also a lot of commercialising activities on hydrolysed formulas.

MarcieMom: *What about the use of free amino acid-based formulas (formulas that do not contain protein chains but the basic amino acids)? Are they an alternative to hydrolysed milk formula? How does it taste and is it better tolerated in infants?*

Professor Hugo: Amino acid formulas are used to treat cow's milk allergy, not to prevent it. These formulas are expensive, and have a bitter taste. Their role in preventing cow's milk allergy seems to be equal to the role of hydrolysed formulas.

MarcieMom: *If the infant has a cow's milk allergy, will partially hydrolysed milk formula result in an improvement in the eczema (despite being partially hydrolysed)?*

Professor Hugo: Partially hydrolysed formulas are not a good treatment of cow's milk allergy. What's better is to give extensively hydrolysed formulas, amino acid formulas, or even soy milk (not goat's milk). Many babies with eczema have no cow's milk allergy and switching to another formula makes no sense.

MarcieMom: *Is there a difference between various partially hydrolysed milk brands in their preventive effects on eczema?*

Professor Hugo: There is no difference between the different partially hydrolysed formulas. In general, the partially hydrolysed HA-milks have similar effects. However, large comparative studies are lacking.

MarcieMom: *What is the age that children can start taking fresh milk instead of milk formula? Does it make a difference if their family has a history of atopy?*

Professor Hugo: Healthy children can start taking fresh milk beyond the age of one year. However, cow's milk by itself has limited nutritional value (except for calcium). Fruits and vegetables should be the main ingredients of a healthy diet in preschoolers.

MarcieMom: *Some parents switch to rice milk once their infants have eczema, but I understand it to be nutritionally deficient. What is your view on rice milk as an alternative to cow's milk?*

Professor Hugo: There are no good studies on the role of rice milk in eczema. In general, rice allergy is very uncommon, and it is better to keep it that way. By massive switching to rice milk in young children, we might induce rice allergy, which would be a disaster for Asia. Don't forget that the role of any milk in children with eczema is minimal.

MarcieMom: *We have largely focused on the mother's diet and lifestyle. Does the health of fathers play a role in the development of eczema in the infant?*

Professor Hugo: I am unable to answer this question, due to a lack of studies.

MarcieMom: *Does probiotic supplementation during pregnancy need to be prescribed by a doctor or can a concerned mother of a baby born into a family with an allergic history buy probiotics off the shelf?*

Professor Hugo: It is better to talk to the physician. Don't experiment during pregnancy or lactation.

MarcieMom: *In your practice in the children's clinic, if you see pregnant mothers who bring their children for consultation diagnosed with eczema would you suggest the mother consider probiotics to prevent eczema in the newborn?*

Professor Hugo: Yes, I do, but only if they plan to breastfeed.

MarcieMom: *For a woman who is already taking probiotic supplements, does she need to stop the supplement when pregnant?*

Professor Hugo: I see no reasons why, provided the probiotics are of good quality.

MarcieMom: *Why are studies on probiotic administration for later weeks of pregnancy? Will probiotics not be useful or harmful in earlier weeks or during midterm pregnancy?*

Professor Hugo: There are no studies on early administration of probiotics during pregnancy. When considering the mechanisms (i.e. the impact on bacterial flora) it seems logical to recommended probiotics late in pregnancy, in hopes of modifying the bacterial flora.

MarcieMom: *I've read that probiotics have resulted in side effects such as infection and bowel tissue damage. Are there individuals with certain conditions who should not take probiotics? Is it then safe for infants?*

Professor Hugo: There are no problems administrating probiotics to pregnant and lactating women, provided they are healthy. This is my only recommendation on administrating probiotics. Not directly to babies. However, a healthy immune system is a condition for prescribing probiotics, in general.

MarcieMom: *There are drinks or yoghurt that are marketed and/or labeled as containing live cultures. Are these effective in eczema prevention?*

Professor Hugo: These drinks are not effective in preventing or treating eczema, but studies are not available.

MarcieMom: *Is there foreseeable harm in moisturising a high-risk baby from birth?*

Professor Hugo: When using suitable moisturisers for babies, no major side effects should be expected.

CHAPTER 6

Eczema Treatment

In this chapter, skin care and treatment options are covered. It is important to note that although there is no cure for eczema, eczema can be controlled. The approach to the treatment of AD should be a **holistic approach**. This not only means that medication is prescribed, but also that advice is given on many aspects of lifestyle, including diet (for children with an underlying food allergy), school and sports activity. In general, it advisable to swim regularly in chlorinated water, followed by extensive moisturising. In children with an underlying house dust mite allergy (common in older children with AD) they are advised to be outdoors as much as possible, and to stay in the bedroom as short as possible (only for sleeping).

Taken together, treatment of atopic dermatitis includes following aspects:

1. Lifestyle changes
2. Diet (in patients with an underlying food allergy)
3. Basic skin care
4. Treatment of eczema patches

Skin Care

As covered in Chapter 2, the skin barrier of eczema patients is defective, with increased skin permeability and increased transepidermal water loss. Moisturising the skin serves to repair the skin barrier, assist the retention of moisture in the skin, reduce the transepidermal water loss and restore the ability of the skin's lipid barrier to retain water. Moisturising has been shown to be able to reduce the frequency and intensity of eczema flare-ups and also reduce the need for topical medication.

Functions of Moisturiser

A moisturiser must therefore possess the following three functions in order to benefit the skin:

i. Increases moisture of skin — Emollients such as structural lipids, mineral oil, lanolin, cholesterol, squalene, stearic acid, linoleic and alpha-linoleic acids increase the moisture of skin by filling in the spaces between corneocytes in the skin barrier. Certain emollients that contain ceramides and natural moisturising factors can temporarily improve the dryness in ceramide-deficient skin.

ii. Prevents transepidermal water loss — Occlusive, acting as a hydrophobic barrier to prevent transepidermal water loss and comprises of lipids such as petrolatum, lanolin, mineral oil, dimethicone/ silicones and zinc oxide. This occlusive function can also reduce the penetration of irritants into the skin.

iii. Attract moisture to the skin — Humectants such as glycerine, sorbital, urea and hyaluronic acids can attract moisture to the skin via enhancing water absorption from the dermis into the epidermis and from the environment.

While it is beneficial to select a moisturiser that can fulfil the above functions, it is equally important to choose one which the patient will use frequently. Factors affecting the likelihood of use include cost and how the patient tolerates the moisturiser, including any irritation or blocked pores after use. In general, it is advisable to use the moisturiser that feels good on the skin of the patient (child), and let the child decide which moisturiser feels the best. Another rule: Use it a lot!

Choice of Lotion or Cream or Ointment

Generally, a lotion is faster to apply but its effect may not be long-lasting. An ointment consists of 80% oil and has better occlusive property but may not be tolerated well for those who sweat often or live in a hot, humid environment. However, for those living in dry conditions or winter, where the humidity falls below 60% and moisture is stripped from the skin, an ointment is often recommended to protect against moisture loss. In areas of higher humidity, a lotion/cream can be used during the day and a cream/ointment applied at night.

How to Moisturise?

Moisturisers should be applied on the whole body, not limited to areas of skin that appear dry or have eczema. Actually, applying a moisturiser on patches of eczema helps very little. Moisturisers should be applied on the dry skin to prevent new eczema patches. It is applied generously and in the direction of hair growth, instead of in a circular motion to prevent accumulation of the moisturiser around hair follicles. It is important to ensure adequate amount of moisturiser is used; for children about 100–200 grams per week and for adults 200–300 grams per week. If using from a tub, be sure to use a clean spatula to prevent contamination with bacteria. Always ensure that the hands are clean before moisturising. For children, moisturising should be done quickly (especially for children who resist moisturising) and parents can teach the importance of moisturising so that the children will apply it on their own in their pre-teens or teen years during school.

When to Moisturise?

Moisturise the skin as often as needed, but always immediately (within three minutes) after a shower or after swimming or bathing. A patient with eczema should not shower for an extended period or do so with hot water, which might reduce moisture and natural oil in the skin. In order to seal the moisture on the skin after a shower, moisturisers (with an occlusive function) should be applied immediately.

Sunscreen

Sunscreen offers protection against the ultraviolet light that can penetrate the epidermis and dermis to induce inflammation and damage the skin. It is to be applied about 30 minutes after moisturising, and about 20 minutes before going into the sun. For those with eczema, sun protection measures are to be taken as eczema lesions that are burnt by the sun can aggravate skin inflammation, resulting in a flare-up. A mineral-based, fragrance-free, non-irritating sunscreen lotion that contains zinc oxide and/or titanium dioxide is recommended. Choose at least SPF30 and take other measures such as wearing long sleeves and a hat to prevent sunburn. Reapply sunscreen every two hours.

Shower

Despite the possibility of drying the skin during a shower, showering daily is essential for (i) good hygiene — washing away oil, dirt, germs, bacterial, fungi and sweat, (ii) removing pollutants, irritants and potential contact allergens, and (iii) removing dead skin or crusted tissue. Water can soften the top layer of skin and make it easier for medication cream and moisturisers to be absorbed. A shower is also relaxing and can relieve stress (which is a trigger for eczema in some individuals).

Shower with a mild, non-soap cleansing product that is non-irritating to the skin. To minimise moisture loss, do not use hot water or shower beyond 15 minutes and avoid scrubbing the skin during the shower. After showering, pat dry instead of rubbing dry. Retain some moisture on the skin and moisturise within three minutes of showering to seal in that moisture.

Baths

There are various types of bath options. For infants, they can be soaked in the bathtub with lukewarm water for 10 to 15 minutes with bath oil or colloidal oatmeal or a mild, fragrance-free cleanser. For those who have skin infection, to prevent bacterial colonisation of the skin, a bleach bath can be prepared two to three times per week, using ¼ cup bleach diluted with 40 gallons of lukewarm water. The concentration of sodium hydrochlorite in the bleach should not be more than 6%. During winter, an emollient bath can be taken where an emulsifying ointment is added to hot water, whisked till creamy and added to the bath. A quick rinse after bath is followed by the same skincare routine after a shower.

Swimming

Regular swimming, three times per week at least, in chlorinated water keeps the bacteria on the skin low and will reduce itch and flare-ups of eczema. It is advisable to moisturise intensively after swimming on a pat-dried skin, to avoid the sun, and to stay only 10–15 minutes in the pool.

Eczema Treatments

Active treatment of eczema is essential, on top of observing the above-mentioned skincare routine. Under-treated eczema patches may result in skin infection (sometimes resulting in general infection) and in permanent scarring of the skin. Therefore, relying on skincare alone is not effective when there is skin inflammation, rashes and flare-ups, as eczema patches do not respond to skin care. The itch-scratch cycle can be controlled when the eczema is treated, and the itch and scratching will be reduced.

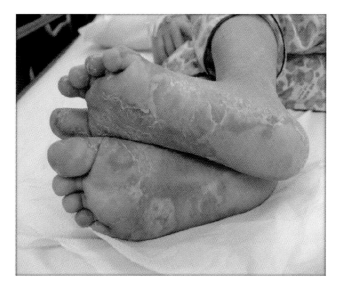

Fig. 6.1   Severe infected eczema.

Medication Cream

Creams prescribed are generally classified into two groups: (i) corticosteroid creams and (ii) non-corticosteroid creams. They should be used as directed by the physician, taking note of the potency of the cream and its frequency and duration of use.

Topical corticosteroids

Topical corticosteroids are prescribed as topical creams that contain corticosteroids which reduce inflammation on the skin. Topical corticosteroids

Table 6.1   Potency of Common Corticosteroids

TOPICAL CORTICOSTEROIDS	RELATIVE POTENCY
Halcinonide 0.1%	Very high
Diflucortolone valerate 0.3%	Very high
Clobetasol propionate 0.05%	Very high
Betamethasone dipropionate — augmented 0.05% — ointment	Very high
Triamcinolone acetonide 0.1%	High
Mometasone furoate 0.1% — ointment	High
Hydrocortisone butyrate 0.1%	High
Fluticasone propionate 0.05%	High
Betamethasone valerate 0.1% — ointment	High
Beclomethasone dipropionate 0.025–0.05%	High
Desoximetasone 0.025%	High
Fluocinonide 0.05%	High
Betamethasone dipropionate 0.05% — cream	High
Flucocinolone acetonide 0.025%	Medium
Mometasone furoate 0.1% — cream	Medium
Methylprednisolone aceponate	Medium
Hydrocortisone valerate 0.2%	Medium
Clobetasone butyrate 0.05%	Medium
Betamethasone valerate 0.05%	Medium
Alclometasone dipropionate 0.05%	Mild
Hydrocortisone (acetate) 0.1–2.5%	Mild
Desonide 0.05%	Mild

are still the cornerstone treatment of eczema patches. They are therefore applied on areas of skin with active lesions and up to a few days after the clearance of skin lesions to reduce inflammation in the underlying layers of the skin. Topical corticosteroids can also be applied on areas of scratch lesions (open skin), scratch wounds and oozing eczema. Potent corticosteroids have also been shown to reduce colonisation of *Staphylococcus aureus*, and have immunosuppressive and vasoconstrictive properties. Corticosteroids of very high potency ought to be avoided in children.

How to apply topical corticosteroids?

Corticosteroids should be applied sparingly, and the finger tip unit of measure (FTU) can be used as a guide. A FTU is the amount of ointment expressed from a tube with a nozzle 5 mm in diameter, from the distal skin crease to the tip of index finger. Similar to applying moisturiser, the hand should be clean before applying. The absorption of corticosteroids can be increased with occlusive treatments, such as emollients or wet wraps. Therefore, patients prescribed with higher than mild potency topical corticosteroids should check with the physician whether it should be applied prior to moisturising and with wet wrap.

High potency topical corticosteroids should be avoided in young children, especially in the face, eyelids, flexures and genital areas. A medium potency cream may be prescribed for such thinner skin regions, followed by a mild potency cream when the eczema patches improve visibly. In general,

Table 6.2 FTU to Treat Various Skin Regions of an Adult

FTU (RANGE)	REGION
6 to 7	Front of trunk
6 to 7	Back of trunk (including buttocks)
5 to 6	Leg
1 to 2	Foot
3 to 4	Arm and forearm
2 to 3	Face, neck and ears
1 to 2	Hand

Table 6.3   FTU to Treat Various Skin Regions of a Child

FTU	REGION
2	Front of trunk
3	Back of trunk (including buttocks)
1.5	Leg
0.5	Foot
1.5	Arm and forearm
1.5	Face and neck
0.5	Hand

the potency of the corticosteroid that is prescribed, the duration and frequency all depend on the severity, location, chronicity and age of the patient. Some physicians may prescribe corticosteroids on areas of skin with frequent eczema flare-ups, even on days when there is no visible flare-up (for usually one to two days per week), also labelled as "pro-active treatment."

A note on corticosteroid phobia

There is increasing fear of using corticosteroids, especially in children. Topical corticosteroids have side effects such as skin thinning, skin irritation, skin discolouration, acne, easy bruising, fragile blood vessels, and excessive hair growth. However, when used as directed, studies have shown that mid-level potency corticosteroids do not result in skin thinning in children over a period of about 10 months. Patients who read of testimonies of side effects of topical corticosteroids should bear in mind that (i) the side effects of misuse should not be confused with those of proper use, and (ii) there are those who stand to gain from steroid phobia, through promoting their steroid-free alternatives. While certain ingredients in topical corticosteroids may trigger hypersensitive reaction for some children, this is not common. Topical corticosteroids should be part of a holistic treatment, along with allergy testing, avoiding allergens, vigilant skincare routine, wet wrap, swimming, and a healthy diet and lifestyle. There is no need to exclude other treatments simply because one is applying corticosteroids.

Topical calcineurin inhibitors (TCI)

TCI are non-steroidal creams that contain calcineurin inhibitors that are T-cell inhibitors: they suppress the effects of the immune system via inhibiting calcineurin that activates T-cells. There are two drug names for TCI creams, namely pimecrolimus and tacrolimus, available by prescription for children above the age of two years, and adults. These creams are recommended as second-line therapy for patients with moderate to severe AD, and usually as part of maintenance therapy for areas of skin such as the face which is thinner and not suited for long-term corticosteroid use. Similarly, using TCI under occlusion should be consulted to prevent excessive absorption into the skin and risk of mild immunosuppression. Some patients report a stinging sensation during the initial period of use of TCI and any discomfort should be reported to the physician. The physician will advise on the duration of use, based on the chronicity of eczema and age of the patient. In rare cases, TCI is not recommended, especially for patients with underlying immune disorders.

Wet wrap

Wet wrap therapy involves two layers of open-weave tubular dressings (inner moist and outer dry) over moisturised skin for added occlusive effect. Wet wrap serves to increase moisture retention, absorption of moisturisers, and limit damage of scratching. The inner moist layer can be dipped in cool or room temperature or lukewarm water, according to the patient's preference. As previously mentioned, steroidal creams should not be applied under a wet wrap without consultating the physician. Wet wrap should be monitored in the presence of skin infection, and also not be continued after the skin recovers and no longer appears dry. In general, children do not like this procedure. Therefore, it is not the first line treatment of AD.

Antihistamines

Antihistamines are available over-the-counter and work through blocking histamine-receptors, thereby avoiding histamine effects, a substance that is released during allergic reactions. Antihistamines have limited use in the treatment of AD, mainly to manage the itch and those that cause drowsiness (e.g. diphenhydramine and hydroxyzine) can help children to have longer period of undisrupted sleep at night. Sedating antihistamines should not be used for long-term, usually for a maximum of two weeks as their effect can be lost.

A note on bedtime

Bedtime is one of the most difficult times of the day to control eczema, in particular scratching and itch, as there is less distraction or activity during bedtime. Sleep, however, is essential for all, especially growing children. The lack of sleep is associated with behavioural issues, a weaker immune system and inability to concentrate. For children, parents can consider establishing a bedtime routine of shower, moisturising (with topical treatment or wet wrap if needed), reading a book, prayer and turning lights off. The room should be kept cool, with air-conditioning if required. Should the air become too dry in the room, a humidifier can be used. The child should go to bed fresh and calm, wearing comfortable cotton pyjamas.

A note on schooling children

For schooling children who cannot get adequate sleep during the night, parents may want to discuss with the school on starting class later. Teachers should be made aware of eczema and how it impacts the child during school, ranging from freshening up after sports, moisturising, choice of material for the school uniform and being mindful that a lack of concentration in class could simply be due to a lack of sleep (and not related to attention disorders).

Oral Medication

Oral medication may be prescribed in severe cases of eczema, and typically can be classified as (i) oral corticosteroids and (ii) immunosuppressants.

Oral Corticosteroids

Oral corticosteroids include medication such as prednisolone and prednisone, which work by suppressing inflammatory reactions. Patients must observe the doctor's prescribed dosage, frequency and duration as it is customised according to the skin condition, weight and health of the patient. Self-varying the dosage can have serious side effects as a heavy dose of prednisolone is used to treat vastly different diseases such as blood cancer and lymphoma.

Long-term use of oral corticosteroids is not advisable due to its potential side effects, including impairment of calcium absorption, thereby slowing down a child's growth, impeding new bone formation and causing the thinning of bones. As oral corticosteroids also lower one's immunity and resistance to infection, it is not advisable to take it over the long-term and care must be taken to avoid those who are ill (especially with chicken pox, measles and shingles) or who have recently taken a live vaccine. Good hygiene should also be practised to prevent infection. Other long-term side effects are high blood pressure, skin thinning, muscle weakness, fluid retention and cataracts.

Immunosuppressants

Common immunosuppressant medications that are used in severe AD are cyclosporine, methotrexate, azathioprine, and mycophenolate mofetil. These medications are used to treat severe, persistent and wide-spread atopic dermatitis that has not responded to other treatments. Similar to corticosteroids, the dosage, frequency and duration of the course is prescribed by a skilled physician and must be adhered to strictly.

Cyclosporine reduces the inflammation on the skin through its suppression of cytokine production by T cells via inhibition of calcineurin. It is important to keep to the prescribed dosage because a higher dosage is meant to treat other conditions, such as the prevention of organ rejection after a transplant. Cyclosporine is not intended for long-term use as there are risks associated with high blood pressure, kidney damage, lymph and skin cancer.

Blood pressure, blood and urine tests are regularly conducted to monitor the creatinine, potassium, blood count, fasting lipid and uric acid levels and the liver function. There are also side effects ranging from mild and short-term ones like nausea to severe effects, such as seizures and vision changes.

The physician may advise on diet modifications, such as (i) avoiding grapefruit which can increase the amount of cyclosporine in the bloodstream, (ii) avoiding foods that are high in potassium as cyclosporine already increases the potassium in bloodstream, and (iii) taking magnesium supplements.

Mycophenolate mofetil is a purine biosynthesis inhibitor, and similar to cyclosporine, also works by lowering the activity of the immune system. Again, it is important to keep to the prescribed dosage because a higher dosage is meant to treat other conditions, such as the prevention of organ (kidney, heart or liver) rejection after a transplant. Mycophenolate mofetil is also prescribed for Crohn's disease.

Mycophenolate mofetil is usually taken before food and should be swallowed whole or in the form of suspension. Blood tests (blood count and chemistry panel) are regularly required to monitor the blood count of white blood cells, red blood cells, and platelets. Swollen gums is a possible side effect and thus patients should take good care of their gums. There is no particular diet to follow, unless directed by the physician.

Methotrexate and azathioprine are antimetabolites that slow down the metabolism of new cells via the inhibition of dihydrofolate reductase (DHFRase), an enzyme involved in the synthesis of DNA, RNA. At higher dosage, they are prescribed to reduce the growth of cancer cells. They are also prescribed for advanced stages of cancer, severe active rheumatoid arthritis, and used to treat severe psoriasis, whereby the formation of skin cells is decreased to prevent the formation of scales. Methotrexate and aza-thioprine have anti-inflammatory properties and also lower the activity of the immune system. Similar to other immunosuppressants, the prescribed dose must be strictly adhered to.

Certain tests may be required to monitor the side effects of antimetabo-lites, such as blood and liver tests. Check with your physician on the amount of fluids to take during the course, as more water may need to be consumed to reduce toxicity in the kidneys. Also check on what sports you can engage in, to prevent cuts or injury. Possible diet medication includes taking folic acid but studies are not definitive in this area as folic acid may also reduce the effectiveness of the antimetabolite medication.

For all the immunosuppressant medication, there is increased susceptibility to skin cancer or increased light sensitivity and thus care must be taken for sun protection and to avoid phototherapy. The reduced resistance to infection also implies avoiding contact with ill persons or persons who were recently vaccinated. Washing hands and observing good hygiene also help to prevent infection. Always let your physician know about the medication and supplements you are taking, as certain medications can interact with the immunosuppressant.

A note on the efficacy of oral medication

The studies on the efficacy of various oral medications are often on a small-scale and difficult to draw conclusions on general efficacy. The important factor for patients to consider is to work with a skilled physician who has experience prescribing such medication and one whom he/she trust to monitor his/her skin condition and reactions to treatments over time.

Antibiotics

Oral antibiotics are prescribed to treat general skin infections while topical corticosteroids containing antibiotics are used on local infected skin lesions. As mentioned in Chapter 2, eczema skin is prone to *Staphylococcus aureus* colonisation, and where the skin is infected, antibiotics treatment is necessary. Due to the increasing resistance of bacteria to common penicillin treatments, antibiotics should be avoided as much as possible. Prevention of infection should be incorporated into skin care routine such as bleach baths, swimming and cleaning the skin with chlorhexidine or other antiseptics (see Chapter 4 "Bacterial Colonisation of Skin").

Photo Therapy

Photo- or light-therapy involves the exposure of the patient to artificial ultraviolet A, ultraviolet B or narrow bands of UVA and UVB. It is to be conducted by a dermatologist, and usually not recommended for children. Light therapy works by reducing inflammation on the skin, but it is also potentially harmful when used for a long time, increasing the risk of skin cancer. It is used with caution for patients who are more susceptible to skin cancer, such as fair skin phenotypes.

Habit Reversal

It is important to break out from the itch-scratch cycle, but for certain patients who have formed the habit of scratching, habit reversal techniques may need to be incorporated into the treatment (apart from treating the eczema lesions). Such techniques include replacing the scratching habit with another habit, and for children, it is helpful to reward them for doing an activity apart from scratching rather than to penalise them for scratching.

Lifestyle

For patients whereby stress has been observed to trigger eczema, it is beneficial to adopt a less stressful lifestyle and also to engage in stress relaxation techniques, such as deep breathing and massage. Exercise can also help to relieve stress and contribute to a healthy body. A positive attitude goes a long way to controlling eczema.

Diet

Except for patients with an underlying food allergy, there is no specific diet that will help with controlling eczema, but it is recommended to eat a balanced diet with plenty of fruits and vegetables. Avoid trans fatty acids present in fast foods and fried foods as higher consumption of these trans fats have been associated with higher incidences of allergic conditions. Supplements have little or no impact on eczema, except for omega-3 supplements, but this needs further study.

Mom Asks, Doc Answers!

MarcieMom: *How can one gauge if a moisturiser is a quality moisturiser?*

Professor Hugo: Moisturisers don't cure, and need to be used several times per day. The most important factor is that the child likes the moisturiser and that the moisturiser doesn't irritate. If these two conditions are fulfilled, one can call the moisturiser a good quality moisturiser for this specific patient.

MarcieMom: *Would a different moisturiser be recommended for someone with visibly dry skin versus one without (both have eczema)?*

Professor Hugo: Yes. If the skin is very dry we will recommend an ointment, but it is important that the patient likes this. If the skin is not dry, moisturising can be limited, and a cream or lotion can be used, according to the preference of child and parents.

MarcieMom: *Will a moisturiser assist the penetration of irritants or allergens into the skin?*

Professor Hugo: This has not been shown. In contrast, moisturising will prevent contact of allergens with the skin and the immune system of the child.

MarcieMom: *How does someone know if his/her skin is deficient in ceramide and therefore, should opt for (the more expensive) ceramide-based moisturiser?*

Professor Hugo: It is impossible to know and not necessary to know. If the skin dryness can be reduced with a moisturiser, and the patient feels better with it, then the moisturiser can be continued. I advise to start with a normal moisturiser, and to test different "normal" moisturisers. In scientific studies, the expensive moisturisers have only very limited advantages, and are often not necessary. Eczema in most children can be controlled with a normal moisturiser.

MarcieMom: *Will continuously using a thicker cream or ointment increase the likelihood of clogged pores? If so, should lotion be rotated with cream/ointment within the day?*

Professor Hugo: This has not been shown in studies. I advise using a moisturiser that the child likes, and to maintain normal skin hygiene. Regular swimming in chlorinated water is healthy for children with eczema for various reasons (sports, staying outdoors, cleaning of the skin).

MarcieMom: *Should an intentional effort be made to wash moisturisers off the skin to prevent an accumulation of previously applied moisturisers?*

Professor Hugo: This is not necessary. I suggest to maintain normal skin hygiene.

MarcieMom: *Do moisturisers trap dirt or bacteria more easily?*

Professor Hugo: This was never shown.

MarcieMom: *Is it advisable to use only one brand of moisturiser, say for the benefits of assessing its impact on the skin as compared to using multiple brands?*

Professor Hugo: It is difficult to give advice on this. If the child is good with a moisturiser, there is no reason to switch, I guess. Moreover, this is a problem that is difficult to study.

MarcieMom: *I've heard of some patients who remarked that switching moisturiser brands seems to show more improvement in the skin compared to sticking to the same brand. Is there a basis for this?*

Professor Hugo: There is no reason or scientific basis for this, perhaps other than the fact that something new can feel better.

MarcieMom: *How thick should the moisturiser be applied? For instance, should we be able to see the moisturiser or not see the moisturiser but a shimmery look on the skin?*

Professor Hugo: It depends on the dryness of the skin. The skin should feel smooth all the time. A shimmery look is not really necessary.

MarcieMom: *Does applying a thick layer of moisturiser lead to waste (i.e. only the part that is next to the skin gets absorbed) or prevent "the breathing of skin?"*

Professor Hugo: A thick layer is not really necessary, but the so-called breathing of the skin will not be disturbed as long as normal hygienic measures are maintained.

MarcieMom: *Can sunscreen lotion be applied as a moisturiser after shower and before heading outdoors? Or should a moisturiser always be applied first?*

Professor Hugo: Yes, if the sunscreen lotion has the functions of a moisturiser; otherwise, apply the moisturiser, wait for 30 minutes, then apply the sunscreen 20 minutes before heading outdoors.

MarcieMom: *There is much difference in opinion with regard to how many times to shower. What is your advice? (I suppose there needs to be some balance between avoiding drying the skin during shower, and an accumulation of too much dirt.)*

Professor Hugo: There are no studies on this, and general advice cannot be given. It all depends on the type of skin and on the need for a shower.

I advise to be restrictive with showering, and not to shower more than twice a day. This becomes unimportant if the skin is not really dry.

MarcieMom: *Can water irritate eczema skin?*

Professor Hugo: Water dries the skin and a dry skin can be itchier. That's why it is advisable to moisturise after water contact.

MarcieMom: *There are many water-related products that suggest changing the water we drink and bathe ourselves in can improve eczema. Are there convincing studies on this?*

Professor Hugo: There have been no good studies on this. There are many theories on eczema, but only a few have been scientifically proven.

MarcieMom: *After using bath oil, is a quick rinse necessary and should the skin be rinsed to the point of not feeling slippery?*

Professor Hugo: When the child is comfortable there is no need for a quick rinse, as long as the skin feels smooth. However, it is a good habit to moisturise after all contact with water.

MarcieMom: *I co-sleep with my child with eczema ever since she became too big to be swaddled, in order to know when she is scratching at night. Do you support co-sleeping? (I've read that the advantage includes reducing stress and bringing comfort to the baby, but the disadvantages include more dead skin for house dust mite and potential for passing on infection.)*

Professor Hugo: I support approaching children with eczema as normal children. Co-sleeping might have psychological disadvantages. The child has to learn to grow up as a normal child. However, temporarily co-sleeping, during periods of flare-up, might have a positive result, but should be assessed individually.

MarcieMom: *Apart from different potency of topical corticosteroids, do they have different structures that work for different types of eczema lesions?*

Professor Hugo: Not really. Corticosteroids mainly differ in potency, not in underlying mechanisms of effectiveness.

MarcieMom: *Is it a process of trial and error in determining which topical corticosteroid is effective?*

Professor Hugo: In a way it is. I suggest starting with low potency corticosteroids, as part of a holistic approach, not as an exclusive treatment. A stronger corticosteroid might be chosen if lesions persist.

MarcieMom: *Is it more effective to use a milder corticosteroid for a longer time or a more potent one for a shorter time? And which one is safer or has fewer side effects?*

Professor Hugo: This should be decided by the treating physician. In general, mild corticosteroids are recommended before switching to more potent ones. In severe flare-ups local corticosteroids become ineffective, even strong ones, and it is better to give a short course (three to five days) of an oral corticosteroid.

MarcieMom: *How long should a patient use the prescribed corticosteroid before giving feedback to the physician of no noticeable improvement in the eczema?*

Professor Hugo: Although corticosteroids are still the cornerstone treatment of eczema patches, they are only part of the holistic treatment of eczema. If all measures are taken appropriately, an effect of corticosteroids should be seen within one week. Most children can be treated with mild corticosteroids; only in severe eczema are more potent corticosteroids necessary.

MarcieMom: *As eczema is periodic (i.e. comes and goes), how does the physician prescribe the right treatment to a child when the eczema is controlled on the day of the consultation, but may flare-up or worsen the very next day?*

Professor Hugo: There is a maintenance treatment (mainly lifestyle and skin care) and a patch treatment. The latter should be adapted to the severity of the lesions, and can be stepped down if there are no active eczema patches.

MarcieMom: *Can one be addicted to topical corticosteroids?*

Professor Hugo: No, this has never been shown in scientific studies. Addiction refers to a psychological problem, inducing a physical problem. Patients will feel better with corticosteroids, but once the disease is under control corticosteroids can be decreased. However, they don't cure eczema, and patches may re-occur.

MarcieMom: *A black-box warning is given for TCI cream. Since its use by physicians in eczema treatment, have there been studies validating or refuting the cancer claims?*

Professor Hugo: TCI creams are safe; only after oral administration is an immune suppression induced, not through topical usage.

MarcieMom: *For wet wrap therapy, I've heard it is possible to overdo it. What does that mean?*

Professor Hugo: Most children with eczema don't need wet wrapping. Moreover, it is not a child-friendly treatment. Overdoing it means that the skin gets damaged or infected, which is unusual under good control.

MarcieMom: *For children with oozing eczema lesions, should it be dried off first before starting wet wrap? If so, how do we dry the oozing skin?*

Professor Hugo: "Wet should be treated with wet." This is a general rule in dermatological treatment. When lesions are oozing they are likely to be infected: wet dressings with antiseptics are recommended.

MarcieMom: *I've read that antihistamine seldom improves eczema or the itch. Is that so? Is it due to the body getting used to the antihistamine or is it because the itch is caused by more variables than just the release of histamine?*

Professor Hugo: Indeed, antihistamines have little or no effect on itch, mainly because histamine does not play an important role in the itch of eczema. Older antihistamines induce drowsiness, and can have an indirect effect on scratching by making the child sleepy. That's why they are used before bedtime.

MarcieMom: *What is the consequence of not following through with an oral corticosteroid or immunosuppressant course?*

Professor Hugo: This can lead to partial treatment, and in a second phase to worsening of eczema, initiating the need for stronger treatments. Oral immunosuppressants and oral corticosteroids should be taken according to the physician's prescription. If not, side effects and worsening of eczema may occur.

MarcieMom: *In general, how many courses of an oral corticosteroid or immunosuppressant will be too much in a year? And when does a physician usually decide if a certain corticosteroid or immunosuppressant is not useful in treating the eczema?*

Professor Hugo: All these medications need to be limited. One course can already induce side effects. Usually we try to be very restrictive with oral immunosuppressants. A few courses per year is the limit: two to four, but it varies individually.

MarcieMom: *What is the safe amount of time to be exposed to light therapy and what spectrum of UV rays are safe?*

Professor Hugo: There are no good studies on this, and therefore we try to avoid UV in children. Only in older children and in cases of severe eczema will this treatment be considered.

MarcieMom: *Will oral antibiotics kill off both good and bad bacteria and make it easier for more bad bacteria to re-colonise?*

Professor Hugo: There is always a selection of bacteria. Usually the strongest will survive, and will have more space to grow. Repeated use of antibiotics will lead to colonisation with multi-resistant bacteria.

MarcieMom: *When would you recognise that a patient needs to work on habit reversal techniques? And how is this carried out in your clinic?*

Professor Hugo: There are no good studies on this. Usually, we will ask the advice of a psychologist in older children with severe eczema. Most children don't need habit reversal techniques. It is all a matter of controlling their eczema.

CHAPTER 7

Atopic Dermatitis in Adults

A lot of the features of atopic dermatitis (AD) in children count for adults. These include features of symptoms, mechanisms, triggers and treatment. AD is mainly a disease of childhood, with the highest prevalence in young children. Most children grow out of AD, dependent on severity and triggers (allergy induces more persistent lesions). Allergic reactions, mainly to house dust mites, seem to be the major maintaining factor, leading to persistence of AD into adulthood. Therefore, AD in adulthood is mainly AD that persisted through childhood, through puberty and into adulthood. Usually adults with AD were former children with severe AD, house dust mite allergy and severe colonisation of the skin with *Staphylococcus aureus*. Other types of AD in adults are late onset AD, which is uncommon, and contact dermatitis, which is more common in adults than in children. Taken together, AD in adults is characterised by severe bacterial colonisation and by an underlying house dust mite allergy. Food allergy is by far less common. Moreover, skin lesions are mainly consequences of past bacterial infection and scarring, resulting in pigment abnormalities (hypo- and hyperpigmentation).

Symptoms

Typically, in adults AD is very itchy, red, and dry, with a high degree of lichenification (the skin is cracked and leathery), skin scarring (hypopigmentation and hyperpigmentation), and signs of skin infection (crusts). AD most frequently appears on the face, neck and extremities, but it can show up in other areas, too. In fair-skinned people, AD lesions may initially appear reddish and then turn brown. Among darker-skinned people, eczema can affect pigmentation, making the affected area lighter or darker.

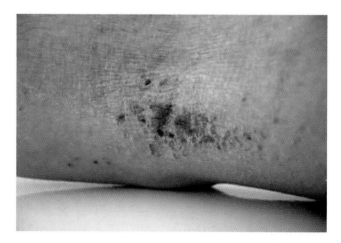

Fig. 7.1   Due to its chronicity, adult eczema is characterised by severe lichenification and crust formation.

Triggers

In adults a large number of non-specific and psychological triggers, such as stress, are able to induce a flare-up of eczema. For some, coming into contact with rough or coarse materials may cause the skin to become itchy. For others, feeling too hot or too cold, exposure to certain household products like soap or detergent, or coming into contact with allergens, such as house dust mites or animal dander (skin or hair) may cause an outbreak. Upper respiratory infections or colds may also be triggers. Food allergy is usually not involved in adult AD, but some patients may suffer from flare-ups after consuming seafood, peanuts or other food.

Treatment

Treatment is similar as in childhood eczema. In adults, the goal of treatment is focused on the relief and prevention of itch. Therefore, moisturising the skin, using lotions and creams (emollients) is a pivotal part of the treatment. These products are usually applied when the skin is damp, such as after bathing or swimming, to help the skin retain moisture. Cold compresses may also be used to relieve itching. Phototherapy is also more in use in adult AD than in childhood AD.

Eczema outbreaks can sometimes be avoided or the severity lessened by following these simple tips.

- Moisturise frequently
- Avoid sudden changes in temperature or humidity
- Avoid sweating or overheating
- Reduce stress
- Avoid scratchy materials, such as wool
- Avoid harsh soaps, detergents and solvents
- Be aware of any foods that may cause an outbreak and avoid them

Approach to Itch in Adult Eczema: Tips to Soothe the Itch

Relieve itch due to dry skin through moisturising

Dry skin tends to be itchy, and therefore, as mentioned in Chapter 6, skin-care, moisturising can increase moisture of the skin, prevent transepidermal water loss and attract moisture to the skin. Moisturisers are the first step in itch control, and a moisturiser has the occlusive function that locks in the skin's moisture. Moisturising is creating an artificial skin barrier, which is necessary as the natural skin barrier in patients with AD is impaired (such as in filaggrin deficiency, and other skin barrier disorders). The key is to moisturise often, especially right after bathing or washing or swimming. It is best to use an unscented moisturiser, because additives and fragrances can irritate the skin.

An ointment consists of 80% oil and has better occlusive property than lotions which are made up of a higher proportion of water. However, not all patients tolerate ointment well, especially for those in hot and humid environments. It is important to use a moisturiser that the patient likes: If the patient likes how the moisturiser feels on the skin, the patient is more likely to use it often.

Relieve itch due to bacterial colonisation

Staphylococcus aureus bacteria produce toxins that act as superantigens and activate inflammatory cells, contributing to inflammatory reactions that trigger itch. Swimming regularly in chlorinated water can keep bacterial colonisation low, followed by moisturising on damp skin after swimming. Diluted bleach bath has the same effect on removing *S. aureus* as well as reducing the likelihood of infection. Adults, similar to children, can have bleach bath two to three times per week, in the same proportion of ¼ cup bleach diluted with 40 gallons of water. The adult can soak for about 10 minutes and then rinse off with water and moisturise immediately after. If the patient's skin is sensitive to bleach, alternatives to removing the *S. aureus* such as swimming or antiseptic can be explored.

Relieve itch through colloidal oatmeal bath

Colloidal oatmeal is able to retain moisture of the skin via its component, avenanthramides that inhibits the release of pro-inflammatory cytokines and histamine. There are commercially available oatmeal bath oils or a pre-packaged oatmeal bath mix can be purchased. Oatmeal bath can be taken daily, each time soaking for about 15 to 20 minutes. Gently pat dry after bath and follow-up with a moisturiser when the skin is still damp.

Relieve itch through cold compress

Cold temporarily stops the transmission of itch through the nerves, and therefore, a cold compress on the skin can relieve itch. An ice pack placed inside a plastic bag or soft towel can form an effective cold compress, usually by holding it against the skin patch that itches. It should be noted that warm compress should not be used as this further dries the skin, increases inflammation and aggravates the skin condition.

Relieve itch by removing triggers

Triggers for eczema have been covered in Chapter 4 and patients should avoid common triggers and also verify specific allergens through allergy testing.

Mom Asks, Doc Answers!

MarcieMom: *Is it more likely for an adult to have eczema if he/she has an allergic disease at childhood (not necessarily childhood eczema)?*

Professor Hugo: Allergy is a risk factor for asthma, rhinitis, eczema, food allergy, and drug allergy. Therefore, a person who is allergic is at an increased risk of developing eczema. However, we don't know why eczema starts in adulthood. Perhaps other triggers are involved, such as viruses, but this has never been proven.

MarcieMom: *Does a family history of parents or siblings outgrowing eczema correlate with whether the child will eventually outgrow eczema?*

Professor Hugo: No, outgrowing eczema is associated with the severity of eczema and underlying triggers. The mechanisms of outgrowing eczema or outgrowing an allergy are still fairly unknown, but might be linked to epigenetic mechanisms (i.e. switch off and switch on of genes).

MarcieMom: *Could diet or lifestyle, say, eating lots of processed food or smoking increase the likelihood of adult-onset eczema?*

Professor Hugo: This is unlikely. If this was the case we would see more adults with eczema. The exact triggers of adult-onset eczema are unknown.

MarcieMom: *Is adult eczema skin more prone to bacterial colonisation than a child's? If yes, why?*

Professor Hugo: Yes, because of the chronicity of the lesions: The longer eczema exists the more colonisation occurs. Keeping the harmful bacteria on the skin low in concentration (without antibiotics) is crucial. Regular swimming in chlorinated water is helpful in most adults with eczema.

MarcieMom: *Are there any common diseases in adults that can trigger eczema? I'm thinking diseases like diabetes, high blood pressure and gastric issues.*

Professor Hugo: No. Eczema is a solitary problem, and is not associated with other diseases, except with being allergic. However, in a number of studies it was shown that allergy is associated with obesity, that seems the only exception.

MarcieMom: *When moderating eczema forums, I frequently see eczema sufferers requesting for help to reduce the skin hypo- or hyper pigmentation. Is this possible at all or will cosmetic procedure have to be taken?*

Professor Hugo: Pigment abnormalities are the consequence of eczema, mainly of suboptimal treatment of eczema. That's why I recommend treating all eczema patches as soon as possible. Once pigment abnormalities have occurred, there is little that can be done. Cosmetic surgery has a very limited effect.

MarcieMom: *In terms of treatment of eczema, is oral medication prescribed more frequently in adults?*

Professor Hugo: Treatment in adults is similar as in children. Usually, we prescribe more sedating antihistamines to suppress itch and to assure a good night's sleep, but only if the patient has sleep disturbances.

MarcieMom: *Is the skin of an adult thicker than that of a child, and should a stronger steroid cream thus be prescribed?*

Professor Hugo: Yes, usually the skin of an adult with eczema is dryer and thicker, because of more severe scarring as a consequence of longer inflammation. Stronger corticosteroids are not required (depends on severity of the eczema). More moisturisation, and the usage of ointments instead of creams is recommended.

MarcieMom: *Does the skin become thinner in old age? Does that mean that an elderly person should not be prescribed a high potency steroid cream or does it not matter as much as skin thinning takes place over many years?*

Professor Hugo: Yes, the skin becomes thinner and of poorer quality (i.e. impaired barrier function) in old age. However, eczema in elderly people is uncommon. The treatment should be adapted to the skin type and the severity of eczema.

MarcieMom: *Children with food allergy are sometimes recommended for repeat allergy tests, is that the same case for adults? Or is the adult's immune system fixed, making repeat allergy testing unnecessary and unlikely to produce different results?*

Professor Hugo: Indeed, in adults allergy is fixed, and repeating allergy tests is less useful. In elderly people (>65–70 years old) severity of allergic reactions goes down spontaneously.

MarcieMom: *For bleach bath, does a stronger or longer bleach bath kill more bacteria? (I'm wondering if an adult can tolerate stronger and longer bleach baths compared to children, and whether that will help remove more S. aureus bacteria.)*

Professor Hugo: This is true in theory, but was never studied. Bleach cannot be too strong as it might irritate the skin.

MarcieMom: *Do the triggers for eczema stay the same throughout a person's life? Or will it stay the same, say, from a certain age?*

Professor Hugo: Allergic triggers are dynamic, especially in early life. Food allergy can be temporarily, while house dust mite allergy usually increases throughout childhood. In adulthood, allergic reactions usually remain stable.

MarcieMom: *Will probiotics help adults with their eczema?*

Professor Hugo: There is no evidence that probiotics are effective in eczema, in children or adults. Only in newborn babies has it been shown that probiotics can prevent the occurrence of eczema, if taken by the breastfeeding mother.

MarcieMom: *Is habitual scratching more prevalent in adults? And if so, how can they seek help?*

Professor Hugo: Habitual scratching is common at all ages, not more common in adults. Holistic treatment of eczema is the best approach. The effectiveness of psychotherapy or behaviour treatment has not been proven.

PART

3

Eczema and Beyond

CHAPTER 8

The Pathophysiology of Atopic Dermatitis

Eczema is a group of diseases or a syndrome with chronic, itchy skin inflammation as its common feature.

Schematically, four major types of eczema can be distinguished:

1. Atopic dermatitis (AD) (eczema in which allergy is involved, the most common type of eczema).
2. Non-atopic dermatitis or constitutional eczema (eczema without allergy).
3. Contact eczema or contact dermatitis (due to direct contact of the skin with foreign substances).
4. Seborrhoeic eczema (with yellowish scaly crust on the scalp, known as cradle cap; its cause is unknown).

Eczema is a dynamic group of diseases. Many children grow out of it and one type of eczema can precede another (usually non-atopic eczema precedes atopic eczema). Moreover, different types of eczema can be present in one patient, such as contact eczema in children with atopic dermatitis.

The exact mechanisms of eczema are still fairly unknown, which is an important reason for the fact that there is still no cure for eczema. However, in most children with eczema, the symptoms can be controlled with symptomatic treatment and appropriate skin care. A causal treatment that prevents or cures eczema is still non-existent. Recently, due to new techniques,

147

important new discoveries on eczema have been achieved. These include: the role of skin barrier abnormalities (such as filaggrin-deficiency), the role of microbiota (germs that transform the skin into an eco-system), and allergy, being a consequence of eczema in most children. However, a lot of knowledge on eczema is still lacking and more studies are needed.

For the moment, the following **hypothetical clinical model** of atopic dermatitis can be constructed, based on age and severity of the lesions (see below). Many of the proposed mechanisms are still hypothetical (not proven), but there are indirect arguments to accept the model, although in the future new knowledge certainly will refine it, or fresh data might shed new light on it.

Hypothetical Model of AD

AD in Early Infancy (Age 1–3 Months) — The Onset of AD

AD is not present at birth but starts during the first weeks or months of life. Children with AD are born with defective skin barrier (genetically determined), such as a filaggrin deficiency or another (non-identified) skin barrier defect. In children with a normal skin barrier, abnormal local immune responses of the skin lay at the onset of eczema. Both abnormalities (skin barrier defect and abnormal skin immune response) can also be present in one patient. Usually, newborns with a skin barrier defect have dry skin from birth.

The abnormal skin barrier defect or abnormal skin immune responses induce abnormal skin colonisation with bacteria (at birth the skin does not contain bacteria, but soon after birth the skin get colonised with a lot of bacteria), which seems to be crucial in the onset of eczema. The abnormal colonisation manifests itself in the lack of diversification of skin microbiota (fewer types of bacteria present, and dominance of *Staphylococcus aureus*), inducing a pro-inflammatory status of the skin, finally leading to skin inflammation (itchy, red skin). The first lesions of inflammation can be due to scratching or rubbing, but are mainly a result of abnormal skin colonisation. Allergic reactions are not present, and the role of auto-antibodies or other triggers (environmental factors, such as viruses) still needs to be elucidated. The child develops non-allergic eczema, with dominance of Th1 lymphocytes in the skin inflammatory lesions (which needs to be proven, as no studies using skin biopsies have been performed).

AD in Early Childhood (Older Infants Aged 3–12 Months and Preschoolers)

Allergic reactions (mainly to a number of foods) appear, mainly in those with severe AD, as a consequence of the defective skin barrier, if the child has an underlying allergic constitution. Allergic sensitisation to food and inhalants occurs mainly transcutaneous (through the skin). Eating or drinking the food is not necessary to develop allergy, as most food is also airborne (i.e. the smelling of food). Because of the skin barrier defects and the chronic skin inflammation, the immune system of the skin is directly exposed to the environment. Direct contact with food or inhalant allergens is responsible for the allergy, leading to a Th2-type of inflammation. Once the allergy has been established any contact (eating, drinking) with the food will result in a flare-up of AD. Common foods involved in AD are egg (number one), cow's milk, soy, and wheat. All other foods are rarely involved in AD (one exception is peanuts, mainly in the USA).

Food allergies in AD are temporary, as most children grow out of their food allergy during the first years of life. Indeed, due to an unknown mechanism most children become tolerant to the foods they were allergic to. For egg it can take up to five to six years, but the other food allergies usually settle earlier. Around the age of one to three years, house dust mite (HDM) allergy starts developing, taking over the role of food allergy. This process is called The Allergic March (switching from one allergy to another). The result is that AD persists, and that its principal maintaining trigger is a HDM allergy.

If children with AD have no atopic constitution, the eczema persists without allergy being involved, and is maintained by mechanical and other (non-identified) non-allergic triggers. The eczema is defined as constitutional or non-allergic eczema. However, this type of eczema usually has a better prognosis and most children will grow out of it before the age of five years, if the lesions are not severe. The more severe the lesions the higher the risk of persistence of the eczema.

AD in Older Children and Adults

In older children, chronic colonisation of the skin by *Staphylococcus aureus* becomes an important maintenance factor of AD. In the meantime, allergic reactions to inhalant allergens become more prominent, especially allergic reactions to the different house dust mites. AD becomes a chronic Th1-mediated inflammation maintained by *Staphylococcus aureus* colonisation (of which the proteins act as super-antigens that maintain inflammation) and by house dust mites. The role of other bacteria (microbiota) is now the subject of intense research. In most food, allergy has decreased, and most older children with AD have no obvious underlying food allergy. If there is a food allergy, this allergy will mainly induce urticaria (hives) and angi-oedema (swelling), having only an indirect effect on AD lesions. Foods involved in older children usually are seafood, nuts, and peanuts. In a number of children auto-antibodies against skin proteins are found in the blood. The role of these antibodies is still largely unknown.

Based on current knowledge of allergy and skin barrier defects it has become obvious that AD is a very complex disease and that a large number of specific features may be involved in its underlying mechanisms. In some children it will be mainly the skin barriers defects that cause the AD, while in others it will be abnormal skin immune responses, mainly allergic reactions or the production of auto-antibodies against the skin proteins. Therefore, AD is considered a SYNDROME (i.e. the atopic eczema/dermatitis syndrome or AEDS), made up of different subtypes, and symptomatic treatment should be individualised, according to the underlying mechanisms and the subtype of AD.

The use of this hypothetical model has *therapeutic impact*, and it is important to position each child in the model, and to find out what phase of AD the child is in.

In phase 1 (onset of AD) the treatment will be focused on moisturising (creating an artificial skin barrier), thereby preventing transcutaneous allergic sensitisation, and on restoring bacterial colonisation by administrating bacterial products early in life (probiotics and prebiotics). In a number of studies it was shown that bacterial products taken by the mother during pregnancy and in combination with breast feeding for six months is able to prevent AD.

In phase 2 treatments will be focused on allergy: avoidance of maintaining food allergens and inhalant allergens.

In phase 3 antiseptic treatments come in, keeping the bad germs (usually *Staphylococcus aureus*) on the skin low. This can be achieved by regular swimming and by regular use of antiseptic solutions, such as bleach, chlorhexidine and zinc-copper sulfate.

In clinical practice, treating eczema is a package that involves changing lifestyle (outdoor activty and swimming), optimal skin care, and symptomatic patch treatment. For those with active eczema, the sun is to be avoided as the sun can worsen the skin inflammation. Should exposure to the sun be too limited, vitamin D supplements can be considered but should be prescribed by the physician.

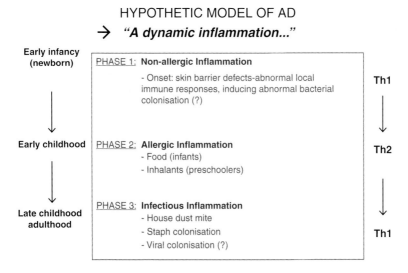

Fig. 8.1   Hypothetic model of AD.

However, a large number of underlying mechanisms are still unknown, and the hypothetical model still largely needs to be studied and proved.

Major deficits in our knowledge on AD are on:

1. The onset of AD
2. The dynamics of AD
3. The role of bacteria
4. The role of auto-antibodies
5. The role of allergic reactions.

Mom Asks, Doc Answers!

MarcieMom: *Is eczema which is under control, i.e. no flare-ups or lesions, considered cured? What is the definition of a condition being cured?*

Professor Hugo: This is a clinical definition, as it is impossible to control (not cure) all microscopic eczema (you cannot perform skin biopsies). Therefore, what we see is what we treat. Usually we accept that eczema is under control if the child has no red patches, little or no itch, and a smooth moisturised skin.

MarcieMom: *How does an abnormal skin barrier defect or abnormal skin immune response induce abnormal skin bacterial colonisation?*

Professor Hugo: This is under study, and the exact mechanisms are still fairly unknown. It has to do with skin receptors, with local cytokine production, and with the buildup of a well-functioning eco-system of the skin, which seems to be impossible in the case of abnormal skin barrier or abnormal immune responses. There are arguments that IL1 secretion is involved, leading to a so-called "pro-inflammatory status."

MarcieMom: *What is the most prevalent way that a food allergen causes a trigger – via consumption, inhaling or contact with the skin?*

Professor Hugo: All routes are possible, and exact data on percentages are not available. In eczema it seems to be mainly through the skin, which is not the case in children with a normal skin. Most babies with severe eczema have an egg allergy, without ever having consumed eggs. More data has become available on this, showing that T-cells from the skin (carrying skin homing receptors) are involved in the allergic reactions.

MarcieMom: *What can be done to lower the likelihood of the Allergic March in children?*

Professor Hugo: Very little, as genes are involved. I advise the following: breastfeeding for six months, probiotics for the mother (last trimester of pregnancy and during breastfeeding) and no extra cleaning of the house or removing of pets. This might have an effect on eczema, far less on allergy.

MarcieMom: *What is viral colonisation in phase 3?*

Professor Hugo: Some viruses are able to induce flare-ups of eczema. The best known example is herpes simplex virus (eczema herpeticum). We suspect that other viruses might be involved, but more studies need to be done on this. The role of viruses in eczema is still largely unknown, but very likely.

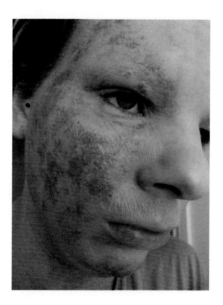

Fig. 8.2   Eczema herpeticum.

MarcieMom: *What about the elderly? Do they undergo a phase when their skin becomes more fragile?*

Professor Hugo: I am not a specialist in elderly medicine, but I know that there is not a lot of research out there on eczema in the elderly. In general, it can be stated that the skin in the elderly is more fragile (thinner), contains more scarring (is more fibrotic) from previous eczema lesions (inflammation), and immune responses have been altered, including a less pronounced IgE-mediated allergy. The latter means that allergic reactions are diminished in the elderly.

MarcieMom: *Is there any possibility that transplants of normal skin flora onto eczema skin can be used to treat eczema?*

Professor Hugo: Transplants of flora are impossible, as skin flora is too dynamic and too specific for each person. However, there are a few studies in adults showing that local applications of "good" bacteria (such as saprophytes) are able to decrease the severity of eczema.

MarcieMom: *Is contact eczema more likely to occur if there is a predisposition to atopic dermatitis?*

Professor Hugo: Yes, in children contact eczema is more common in those who already have eczema (atopic eczema or constitutional eczema). In adults contact eczema is more a unity on itself, occurring without the existence of previous eczema.

CHAPTER 9

Things that Don't Work

Many factors come into play when controlling the different types of eczema. What has been covered in this book will assist parents, caregivers, and physicians in approaching eczema, from its diagnosis to avoiding the known triggers for eczema, and applying the appropriate skincare and treatment. However, given that eczema is a chronic condition that is not curable, there are patients and parents who try alternative treatments in the hope of curing eczema. From experience, certain possible reasons that motivate patients to try other treatments are:

1. No identification of triggers for eczema — Some patients may not know about allergy testing or have no resources to go for an allergy test. As a result, they are unable to take steps to avoid the allergens (food or inhalants), and therefore constantly have eczema flare-ups.

2. Incorrect information about skincare and treatment — There are many misunderstandings in relation to skincare, for instance, that applying emollients will stop your skin from breathing, or that, there is no need to moisturise when there is no eczema flare-up. Similarly with regard to treatment, many fear applying corticosteroid creams, and as a result, the eczema remains untreated.

3. Skin infection — It is also possible that the skin with eczema lesions is colonised or infected with either bacteria or fungi, and therefore, without first treating the skin infection, further treatment has limited efficacy. Keeping the skin clear from infections (i.e. keeping skin germs low) is part of the treatment of eczema. Usage of antiseptic treatments should be routine, while antibiotics have to be avoided, if possible.

4. Minimal improvement in eczema — Every individual responds differently to treatment, and there are patients, parents and caregivers who are informed and follow the appropriate skincare and treatment, but still find that the eczema results in an unacceptable quality of life, mainly caused by the itch, the skin appearance or the lack of sleep and constant scratching.

5. Unrealistic expectation of controlled eczema — Another possible reason is that the patient or parent may hold unrealistic expectations of what eczema under control ought to be; some may expect normal skin with no flare-ups or no scratching and aim to achieve so through alternative treatment.

For many possible reasons, patients may decide to try non-conventional treatments. Below is a list of those treatment and explanations why such treatments or "cures" are ineffective.

1. Dietary supplements — As eczema is a skin condition attributed to a defective skin barrier and abnormal skin immune responses, and not to a nutritional deficiency, dietary supplements have not been proven capable of improving eczema.

2. Diet with minimal food groups — The elimination diet has been covered in *Chapter 4: Triggers for Eczema*, which involves removing suspected foods for a few weeks or months (always at the direction of the physician), then adding back the foods one at a time to observe which food is triggering hypersensitive reactions. However, this is sometimes misunderstood as eating as few foods as possible in order to reduce eczema flare-ups due to food allergy. This will not work if there is no food allergy, as it is possible that the eczema flare-up is not due to a food allergy but to allergy to inhalants or to non-allergic triggers. Even when food allergy is involved, only the food that has been confirmed by allergy testing should be avoided in order to not compromise the nutritional needs, in particular those of a growing child.

3. Intentional exposure to allergens — The other school of thought is to intentionally expose the patient to the suspected allergen. This should

not be attempted because (i) certain exposure may lead to severe allergic reaction, including anaphylactic shock, and (ii) there is no proven study that intentional exposure to allergens can reduce future allergic reaction. Moreover, the mechanism of how a child can "outgrow" an allergen is not known. Exposing a patient to an allergen can make the allergy worse.

4. Intentional exposure to bacteria — Due to the Hygiene Hypothesis, which claims that the increase of allergy during the last 30 years is, at least partially, due to a decreased bacterial load, some parents misunderstand the Hygiene Hypothesis and may intentionally expose their child to more dirt or reduce hygiene practice. This again is not proven, and moreover, increases the risk of bacterial colonisation of the skin, which may lead to skin infection and reduce the efficacy of treatment.

5. Alternative treatments — Acupuncture, homeopathy, Traditional Chinese Medicine and other "natural" remedies are often marketed as being able to cure eczema. There are limited studies on these and therefore it is impossible to conclude that they are effective in treating eczema. Moreover, a lot of (expensive) diagnostic tests are promoted on the Internet. These alternative diagnostic tests (including for food allergy) have no value.

As it is not possible to insist that patients not try alternative treatments, below are a few guidelines for patients and parents:

1. Assess the level of support of the treatment — If multiple clinical trials have been conducted in different (independent) centres and accepted by the international dermatology community, this indicates a safe treatment. Do not be afraid to ask for supporting studies, or ask to see the ingredient list of the prescription to ensure that it does not contain harmful toxins or heavy metals. If a treatment is marketed based on customers' testimonials, you may wish to find out from independent users who comment on the treatment on the Internet.

2. Review the credentials of the company — Find out when the company was established, who established it, their manufacturing facility and

their safety process, in particular for companies that produce emollients. Find out more on the ingredients and whether they are produced in a non-contaminated environment.

3. Review the ingredient list — Whether it is an oral medication or supplement, or creams to be applied, ask for the list of ingredients and make sure there are no harmful substances in it or allergens that might induce symptoms.

4. Inform your physician — If you would like to try a treatment and are already seeing a doctor for your eczema, it is good to ask and update the doctor of the treatment.

5. Be discerning of photographs and testimonials — Questions you can ask yourself are: "Is this photograph showing eczema?", "Are the before and after photographs credible?", "Does the customer giving the testimonial have a vested interest?"

6. Patch test and monitor results — If you are trying a new cream on the skin, test it on a small patch of skin. Ask what to expect during and after the treatment and what the follow-up plan is.

As a concluding thought on this chapter, patients or parents are urged to focus on proven treatment and to apply the appropriate skincare routine. It is important to find a doctor you can trust and communicate with, as likely, you will be seeing the doctor more than once. Do not turn to unconventional treatment simply because you do not trust your existing doctor; it may be more risky to do so. Should you like to try an alternative treatment, be discerning and do not be afraid to question it as you would question a conventional treatment.

Finally, don't forget: eczema is still not curable; therefore, it is also big business, and many (bad) people want to profit from it. Not everything you read on the Internet is true, and there are many websites giving wrong information on diagnostic tests and treatments for eczema.

Mom Asks, Doc Answers!

MarcieMom: *How do you usually handle questions from patients on skin-care or treatment? Do you encourage patients to ask questions, no matter how unscientific they may seem?*

Professor Hugo: It is important to have a good relationship with parents and patients. I try to find out all alternative treatments they are using — to be sure, most try out many treatments. I focus on the dangers of using non-proven treatments and on a scientific approach. And, finally, I ask them not to believe everything that is posted on the Internet and to be very critical, as there is no cure for eczema.

MarcieMom: *When prescribing corticosteroids, how do you handle the steroid phobia? Would you explain the side effects upfront so that patients will not be worried when they go home and search the Internet for information?*

Professor Hugo: I fully explain the effects and the possible side-effects of the different corticosteroids, especially of oral corticosteroids. Once the lesions have improved I switch to corticosteroids of lower potency. Low-potency corticosteroids, used two times per day and only on active eczema patches, have little or no side effects.

MarcieMom: *How does a parent know if a child's skin is infected? Is a visit to the doctor required to be prescribed anti-bacterial or anti-fungal cream or will swimming or cleaning with chlorhexidine be sufficient?*

Professor Hugo: It is impossible to know if a skin is colonised, unless skin cultures are taken. However, from many studies we know that most eczema is colonised from early age (beyond infancy). Therefore, it is part of the routine treatment to keep colonisation under control, by using antiseptics or by recommending regular swimming in chlorinated water.

Usage of antibiotics should be very restricted and only on obviously infected lesions (not to treat skin colonisation).

MarcieMom: *Why is it that for some children and teenagers, their eczema cannot be controlled despite following the appropriate skincare and treatment? Is it the changing immune system or hormones?*

Professor Hugo: There are many reasons, including not identifying the triggers, wrong diagnosis, high skin colonisation, or suboptimal compliance to the treatment (mainly due to environmental triggering). For each patient the reasons have to be found, and some patients with severe eczema need systemic immunosuppression, but this is only a small group.

MarcieMom: *What is a reasonable expectation that parents should have of what eczema under control is like for their children? Personally, I consider not having to use mild corticosteroid for more than once a week, a reasonable amount of sleep, and being able to go to school and participate in family activities as having eczema under control.*

Professor Hugo: I agree. The child should have a normal and happy life, and only using escape treatment (patch treatment) a few times per week.

MarcieMom: *While we know that diet alone will not improve eczema, should patients with eczema make an effort to eat more of certain food groups or reduce foods that promote inflammation like those with trans fats and sugar?*

Professor Hugo: This is still under research, and too early to recommend. The impact of a diet seems to be very low, and only suggested in large groups of patients, such as in the ISAAC study (not in an individual patient). These are statistical significant results, not clinical significant results — and there's a huge difference between the two. The conclusion of the studies on diet is that causal association is not yet shown.

MarcieMom: *Suppose a company does provide the results of their trials or studies to patients. How does one assess if the study or trial is reliable?*

Professor Hugo: This is difficult, especially for persons without medical training. Companies have their own specialists in the field. Usually I look at methodology, patient selection, statistics, and study design. Also, we must realise that a company will not publish a study if the results are negative. The best are independent studies, performed in different university centres, showing similar results. Be careful with "spectacular results." Usually, these are not true.

MarcieMom: *What should patients avoid when deciding on products?*

Professor Hugo: Any product that irritates the skin should be avoided. Moreover, it is advisable to use local treatments (moisturisers, creams, antiseptics) that have been proven to be safe and effective. Don't experiment!

MarcieMom: *There are many topical products which are made by individuals. What is the risk of buying a cream made by someone from their home?*

Professor Hugo: I recommend not to try out creams on your child, and to stick to creams that have been proven to be safe and effective.

MarcieMom: *What can be done to safeguard patients from undeclared active ingredients in alternative medications?*

Professor Hugo: Same answer: Don't experiment with your child and use only products that have been studied on efficacy and safety. Usually, "alternative" medications are not well studied, especially in children.

MarcieMom: *Are there any ingredients that should be avoided, not because they harm the eczema as such, but because they may work against the active ingredients being used in conjunction with each other?*

Professor Hugo: This has not been studied. Usually, I recommend sticking to medications that have been studied.

MarcieMom: *How do you normally respond when a patient asks you about an unconventional treatment that he/she is contemplating? Should the patient decide to give it a go and continue to see you for consultation, does knowing there is another treatment affect how you treat the patient?*

Professor Hugo: I stick to science. If you allow non-scientific products or approaches to come in, everybody is right and risks for all kinds of side effects increase.

MarcieMom: *What alternative therapies don't work?*

Professor Hugo: One has to consider all medications that have not been studied (i.e. no scientific data) as ineffective and potentially dangerous. Don't use them!

MarcieMom: *I always believe that no known side effect in an alternative treatment does not mean there is no side effect. These treatments are usually not subject to as many studies as conventional treatments. What are the possible side effects that patients should look out for in a topical treatment versus an oral medication?*

Professor Hugo: I suggest not to try out treatments that have insufficient data on effectiveness and safety. If not, anything can happen.

MarcieMom: *How do you build trust and relationship with your patient?*

Professor Hugo: In a nutshell: be honest, don't lie, and focus on limitations.

CHAPTER 10

Future Research on Atopic Dermatitis

In recent years, a lot of progress has been achieved in our understanding of allergic reactions and allergic diseases, including atopic dermatitis (AD). However, a lot of research still needs to be done to be able to answer more questions, including two crucial questions concerning AD: **how to prevent it and how to cure it**, as the processes of both onset and outgrowing AD are still fairly mysterious. Giving a complete overview of all new findings is beyond the scope of this book, and can be found in recent review articles on allergy and AD. In this chapter, insights of important and specific topics that are now under intense research are summarised.

Allergic reactions involved in AD seem to be more complex than was initially postulated. In the past, it was accepted that allergy was merely an interplay between a genetic constitution and allergen exposure. Now we know it is more complex, as other players modulating the immune system are involved. Among them are viruses and microbiota (or microbioma, being the genomes of the micro-organisms that reside in an environmental niche, such as the skin). Both have an important role in the functioning of the immune system and in the severity and type of allergic reaction. Another important mechanism that is now under study and that seems to be involved in allergy is epigenetic mechanisms (epigenetics), being the dynamics of gene expression (switching off and on of genes), which is under the influence of the environment (role of pollution, processed foods, etc). Methylation of genes is able to switch off gene activity and is involved in eczema, and might be induced by environmental factors, such as smoke, pollution, stress, and infectious agents.

Other specific important findings in AD are new findings on the role of the skin barrier, including the role of filaggrin, and the fact that sensitisation to foods can occur through a defective skin (transcutaneous). The role of other skin barrier proteins in AD is now a field of intense research.

Top Five New Research Findings in AD

1. The role of microbiota — microbioma.
2. The role of early environmental exposure (allergens, viruses, bacteria).
3. The role of transcutaneous sensitisation in food allergy in AD.
4. The role of the skin barrier (filaggrin and other skin barrier proteins).
5. The role of epigenetics (gene regulation).

The Future Approaches and Future Treatments

There are still numerous issues of AD and allergic diseases in children that need to be explored, as current knowledge is still limited. The topics can be divided into diagnostic topics (also covering mechanisms and pathophysiology) and management topics (focusing on prevention, control and cure of allergic diseases). Briefly, the following are the main fields that need to be studied in the near future.

On the diagnosis of AD

1. We need to learn more about the **genetics** and the impact on the environment on gene expression (epigenetics), especially the role of the environment during pregnancy and in early life. This will enable us to identify risk factors more adequately, and to start treatment (or prevention) early in life.
2. We need to know more about the role of **micro-organisms** (microbioma), including the role of *Staphylococcus aureus*, in the onset, maintenance and outgrowing process of AD. The onset of AD seems especially

to be a consequence of abnormal bacterial colonisation (decreases ability of diversification). The question is still why? And what is the role of skin barrier proteins?

3. We need to know more about the exact role of the different **skin barrier proteins and local immune responses** in AD.

4. We need to know more about the many **phenotypes of AD**. Why is it that some children are very allergic and yet have no symptoms at all? Why is it that other children with only a mild allergy will develop severe AD or severe asthma? Why is it that children of the same parents can show different types of allergy?

5. We need to know more on the role of the **environment** on AD (role of pollution, heat, processed foods, allergens) and on the role of **psychological** factors.

6. We need to know more on the **natural evolution** of AD in children. What makes AD persist and why do a large number of children grow out of it? What makes a child grow out of AD (the mechanisms of growing out of a disease)? Once we know the mechanisms we might start developing a curative treatment.

On the management of AD

1. We should develop better controller treatments with high efficacy and no side effects. Furthermore, all controller treatments should be child friendly, easy to administer, cheap, and accessible to every child, worldwide.

2. We should develop treatments that can cure children with allergy, such as immunotherapy (example: Sublingual Immunotherapy, "SLIT"). These treatments should have a long-lasting effect, and without side effects on the immune system of the child. Furthermore, these treatments should fulfill the same conditions as any controller treatment (see above).

3. We should develop strategies to prevent AD in newborns (or families) at risk for AD.

Prevention of AD: "What Can I Do to Prevent My Newborn Baby from Developing AD or Becoming Allergic?"

Preventing AD or prevention of allergic sensitisation in a healthy new-born is called *primary prevention*. Often, allergic parents consult a doctor, asking him to prevent allergy from occurring in their healthy new-born, and often the doctor will have to admit that this is a very difficult task, mainly because allergy is a genetic disease and not much can be done by trying to manipulate the environment. However, recently a number of important observations have been performed, showing that at

Table 10.1   Primary Prevention Strategies and Their Outcomes

STRATEGY	OUTCOME (LONG-TERM)
Prolonged breastfeeding	Breastfeeding for four to six months is the best. It is useful for the child's health and may prevent AD and allergy in early life. However, there is no clear benefit for the development of inhalant allergies later in childhood that are involved in allergic asthma and allergic rhinitis.
Hydrolysed formula feeding (HA-milks)	Partially hydrolysed formulas in young at-risk infants prevent the incidence of food allergy and AD up to the age of three to five years, but have no benefit if given beyond the sixth month of life. Partially hydrolysed formulas have zero to little effect in the treatment of AD. In children with cow's milk allergy (as a causative factor in AD), totally hydrolysed formulas are advised.
Delayed introduction of solid foods	There is no evidence that delayed introduction of solid food after six to eight months of life is useful in preventing AD or food allergy.
Avoidance of indoor inhaled allergens	Contradictory results. Reduction of exposure to indoor allergens (house dust mites) might even increase the risk for allergy and asthma.
Avoidance of pollution and smoke	Pollution and smoke avoidance is mandatory to maintain respiratory health, and may be effective in reducing the risk of asthma and allergy.

least AD and allergic manifestations can be partially prevented or postponed.

Until recently, primary prevention was mainly based on the assumption that allergen avoidance (foods and inhalants) is the most effective measure to prevent allergic sensitisation and its consequences. Based on this, studies on primary prevention measures have specifically targeted nutrition and environmental control in newborn babies.

The most striking results on primary prevention have been shown for prolonged breastfeeding and for avoidance of pollution and smoke.

Apart of this, other measures, such as hydrolysed formulas or late introduction of solid foods showed far less convincing results. Furthermore, avoidance of inhalant allergen exposure showed contradictory results, even leading to increased sensitisation to these allergens.

The role of bacterial products in primary prevention is now intensively studied. Most studies on probiotics, prebiotics and synbiotics show positive results on AD (not on allergy), if started during pregnancy and given in combination with breastfeeding. Formulas containing bacterial products are far less effective.

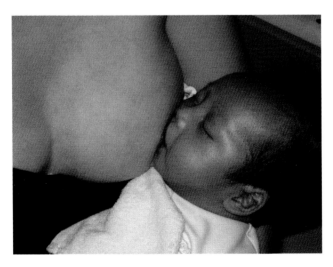

Fig. 10.1   Breastfeeding remains the best way of preventing atopic dermatitis.

In conclusion, many more studies are needed on primary prevention and on the early events of AD, addressing the following issues:

1. The mechanisms of the initiation of AD in newborns (which molecules are responsible for the start of allergy).
2. The exact profiles of the genes that are involved in AD to different allergens (foods, inhalant allergens).
3. The exact role of bacterial products in the treatment of AD (probiotics, prebiotics, and synbiotics), including the best type of bacterial product, best dose, and best window of administration.
4. The exact role of early allergen exposure, including whether high allergen exposure is able to induce tolerance to allergens (including the role of early administration of immunotherapy, including SLIT).

Allergic Diseases in the Future: Aims for Approach

— All children with AD worldwide should receive optimal and early treatment, enabling them to have a healthy life.
— Because of the high prevalence of AD and allergy, every newborn baby should be screened for allergy. According to the risk, optimal primary prevention should be able to decrease the development of subsequent allergic disease.

Mom Asks, Doc Answers!

MarcieMom: *With more factors surrounding AD, does it make it more or less difficult to treat eczema?*

Professor Hugo: Eczema is a very complex syndrome (group of diseases). For each patient the underlying mechanisms should be unraveled, leading to a tailored treatment. The more we know about the mechanisms, the better we can treat eczema. Therefore, I believe that by identifying more of the factors involved, it becomes less difficult to treat the lesions.

MarcieMom: *Should current treatments take into account new developments in eczema research, even when they are not "finalised" yet?*

Professor Hugo: I prefer to adapt or use new treatments only when the data has been proven. For new treatments, they should have been proven to be safe and effective before I start using them in clinical practice.

MarcieMom: *What is Sublingual Immunotherapy or SLIT? Is this a common treatment for children?*

Professor Hugo: SLIT is now very much under study, and the first results in certain specific types of eczema are encouraging. SLIT means daily administration of the allergen under the tongue (as a liquid) — sublingual, means "under the tongue" — and is now in use in patients with allergic asthma and allergic rhinitis, but not yet for eczema. Especially for house dust mite allergy this treatment can become a solution. The first trials on SLIT in food allergy (mainly peanuts) and in eczema are now ongoing, and look promising.

MarcieMom: *Is phenotyping going to offer a way forward for developing new treatments?*

Professor Hugo: This is possible, but not certain for the moment. It is possible that a better tailored treatment will be offered if more features of eczema have been characterised.

MarcieMom: *Would research into non-compliance help?*

Professor Hugo: Sure, and not only in eczema. Compliance is a huge problem in all chronic diseases, and difficult to study.

MarcieMom: *With so much that we do not know of eczema, does it then lend support for parents to try out unconventional treatment?*

Professor Hugo: A short answer: Don't experiment with your child, stick to proven treatments!

CHAPTER 11

Conclusion

Eczema is a group of chronic skin diseases of which atopic dermatitis (i.e. eczema in which allergy is involved) is the most common type. Recent data from epidemiological studies suggest that there is an increase in the prevalence of AD, especially in developed countries. Due to its characteristics, in particular itchy skin inflammation leading to sleep disturbances and impaired school results, and skin abnormalities (rashes in the face), many children and patients with eczema experience considerable impact on their quality of life, including a low self-esteem.

Unfortunately, there are still many aspects of eczema that are unknown. While a lot of progress has been made in making a correct diagnosis, skincare and symptomatic treatment, prevention and cure of eczema are still impossible.

The authors hope that the book has contributed to the understanding of eczema, which might improve approach by patients, parents and caregivers to this complex disease. Moreover, no questions by any mother of a child with eczema have been dismissed, as the authors desire to keep their conversation authentic and reflective of real-life questions of patients and parents. A lot of work (research) still needs to be done, but during the last years, due to intense research, our understanding of eczema has very much improved. Expectations are high to further unravel this disease and to offer prevention and a cure in the near future.

Appendix A

Daily Food Journal

Parents may wish to keep a food journal to note reactions (if any) to foods for communication to your physician.

MEAL	FOOD AND DRINKS	REACTION (ESTIMATED START TIME TO END)
Breakfast		
Mid-morning snack		
Lunch		
Afternoon snack		
Dinner		
Supper		

Appendix B

Checklist to Alternate Caregiver

It is likely that parents will need to prepare a checklist to guide the skincare routine for a child with eczema. This sample checklist does not include allergy avoidance or the use of epi-pen.

SKINCARE ROUTINE	SKINCARE POINTERS	TIME
Moisturising	Usually at every diaper change or approximately once in the morning, afternoon and evening (inclusive of immediately after shower).	
	Use only the emollient provided.	
	Apply in a downward motion.	
	Moisturise even when the skin looks good.	
	Do not moisturise over sweaty skin.	
Shower	Usually one to two times a day, including once before bedtime.	
	Do not shower with hot or warm water, and not beyond 15 minutes, as this will dry the child's skin.	
	Use only the bath oil/lotion and shampoo provided.	
	Pat dry, do not rub dry, retaining a little wetness on the skin.	
	Moisturise immediately after shower.	
	If child's eczema is triggered by sweat, shower the child if there is sweating after outdoor play (and apply sunscreen before going outdoors).	

(Continued)

	(*Continued*)	
SKINCARE ROUTINE	SKINCARE POINTERS	TIME
Treatment*	Clean the eczema skin patch with chlorhexidine using a cotton pad.	
	Apply sparingly the topical corticosteroid provided.	
	Continue to apply the topical corticosteroid for one to three days after the eczema has subsided.	
	Do not apply more than twice a day.	

*If topical corticosteroids only need to be applied once a day, it is best to be performed by the primary caregiver/parent to ensure that the right amount is used.

References

1. INTERNET SITES

There is a lot of information on allergy and eczema in children on the internet. Some sites are very good, giving high level scientific information. However, a considerable number of sites are not good: they have commercial purposes, give wrong information or focus on new "miracle" treatments, without any scientific evidence. We all should be aware of this! The following sites are recommended for further reading. Most of them are official sites of international or national medical organizations:

On Allergy:

American Academy of Allergy Asthma and Immunology (AAAAI): http://www.aaaai.org/

Asia Pacific Association of Allergy, Asthma and Clinical Immunology (APAAACI): http://www.apaaaci.org/

Asia Pacific Association of Pediatric Allergy, Respirology and Immunology (APAPARI): http://www.apapari.org/

Children's Allergy Network "I CAN!" (Singapore) http://www.ican.com.sg

European Academy of Allergy and Clinical Immunology (EAACI): http://www.eaaci.org/

Food Allergy Research & Education (FARE): http://www.foodallergy.org/

World Allergy Organization (WAO): http://www.worldallergy.org/index.php

On Eczema:

American Academy of Dermatology (AAD): http://www.aad.org/

DermnetNZ: http://www.dermnetnz.org/
National Eczema Association (NEA): http://www.nationaleczema.org/
National Eczema Society: http://www.eczema.org/
Nottingham Support Group for Carers of Children with Eczema (NSGCCE):
   http://www.nottinghameczema.org.uk
Mei's website on eczema, entitled "Eczema Blues": http://eczemablues.com/
Website for this book: http://EczemaQnA.com
PUBMED: is an important site on which all medical literature can be found,
   using key words. Just type in a key word and you will find a lot of good
   information on allergic diseases in children. http://www.ncbi.nlm.nih.
   gov/sites/entrez

2. TEXTBOOKS

1. Adkinson NF, Yunginger JW, Busse WW, *et al.* (eds.) (2003) *Middleton's Allergy. Principles and Practice, 6th ed.* Mosby, Inc.
2. Warner J and Jackson WF (eds.). (1994) *Color Atlas of Pediatric Allergy.* Mosby — Year Book, Europe Limited.
3. Delves P, Martin S, Burton D and Roitt I. (2006) *Roitt's Essential Immunology, 11th ed.* Blackwell Publishing.
4. Holgate ST and Church MK. (1993) *Allergy, 1st ed.* C.V. Mosby.
5. Ring J, Przybilla B and Ruzicka T (eds.). (2005) *Handbook of Atopic Eczema, 2nd ed.* Springer.
6. Williams HC (ed.). (2000) *Atopic Dermatitis: the Epidemiology, Causes and Prevention of Atopic Eczema, 1st ed.* Barnes and Noble (2000).
7. Van Bever H. (2009) *Allergic Diseases in Children: the Science, the Superstition and the Stories.* World Scientific.

3. ARTICLES IN MEDICAL JOURNALS

A large number of articles have been published on eczema. Most can be found on PubMed (website: http://www.ncbi.nlm.nih.gov/pubmed). Here, key references are mentioned, according to subject.

1. Review Articles

Rancé F, Boguniewicz M, Lau S. (2008) New visions for atopic eczema: an iPAC summary and future trends. *Ped Allergy Immunol* **19** (19): 17–25.

Akdis CA, Akdis M, Bieber T, *et al.* (2006) Diagnosis and treatment of atopic dermatitis in children and adults: European Academy of Allergology and Clinical Immunology/American Academy of Allergy, Asthma and Immunology/ PRACTALL Consensus Report. *J Allergy Clin Immunol* **118**: 152–169.

Bieber T. (2008) Atopic dermatitis. *N Engl J Med* **358**: 1483–1494.

Van Bever HP, Llanora G. (2011) Features of childhood atopic dermatitis. *Asian Pac J Allergy Immunol* **29**: 15–24.

2. Epidemiology of Eczema

DaVeiga SP. (2011) Epidemiology of atopic dermatitis: A review. *Allergy Asthma Proc* **33**(3):227–34.

Tan TN, Lim DL-C, Lee BW, Van Bever HP. (2005) Prevalence of allergy-related symptoms in the second year of life. *Ped Allergy Immunol* **16**: 151–6.

Stensen L, Thomsen SF, Backer V. (2008) Change in prevalence of atopic dermatitis between 1986 and 2001 among children. *Allergy Asthma Proc* **29**: 392–396.

Asher M.I., *et al.* (2006) Worldwide time trends in the prevalence of symptoms of asthma, allergic rhinoconjunctivitis, and eczema in childhood: ISAAC Phases One and Three repeat multicountry cross-sectional surveys. *Lancet* **368**: 733–43.

Odhiambo JA, Williams HC, Clayton TP, *et al.*, and the ISAAC Phase Three Study Group. (2009) Global variations in prevalence of eczema symptoms in children from ISAAC Phase Three. *J Allergy Clin Immunol* **124**(6): 1252–1258.

Williams H, Stewart A, von Mutius E, *et al.*, and the International Study of Asthma and Allergies in Childhood (ISAAC) Phase One and Three Study Groups. (2008) Is eczema really on the increase worldwide? *J Allergy Clin Immunol* **121**(4): 947–954.

Kay, J., *et al.* (1994) The prevalence of childhood atopic eczema in a general population. *J Am Acad Dermatol* **30**: 35–39.

3. Symptoms of Eczema

Spergel JM and Paller AS. (2003) Atopic dermatitis and the atopic march. *J Allergy Clin Immunol* **112**: S118–127.

Gelmetti C and Colonna C. (2004) The value of SCORAD and beyond. Towards a standardized evaluation of severity? *Allergy* **59**(78): 61–65.

4. Contact Dermatitis

Simonsen AB, Deleuran M, Mortz CG, Johansen JD, Sommerlund M. (2013) Allergic contact dermatitis in Danish children referred for patch testing — a nationwide multicentre study. *Contact Dermatitis* Sep 19. doi: 10.1111/cod.12129.

Simonsen AB, Deleuran M, Johansen JD, Sommerlund M. (2011) Contact allergy and allergic contact dermatitis in children — a review of current data. *Contact Dermatitis* 65(5): 254–65.

5. Eczema in Adults

Silverberg JI, Hanifin JM. (2013) Adult eczema prevalence and associations with asthma and other health and demographic factors: A US population-based study. *J Allergy Clin Immunol* Oct 3. pii: S0091–6749 (13) 01366-3.

Na CR, Wang S, Kirsner RS, Federman DG. (2012) Elderly adults and skin disorders: common problems for nondermatologists. *South Med J* 105(11):600–6

6. Underlying Mechanisms (Skin Barrier Disorders, Allergy, and Role of Staphylococcus Aureus and Microbiota)

Elias PM, Hatano Y, Williams ML. (2008) Basis for the barrier abnormality in atopic dermatitis: Outside-inside-outside pathogenic mechanisms. *J Allergy Clin Immunol* **121**: 1337–1343.

Cork MJ, Robinson DA, Vasilopoulos Y, *et al.* (2006) New perspectives on epidermal barrier dysfunction in atopic dermatitis: Gene-environmental interactions. *J Allergy Clin Immunol* **118**; 3–21.

Leung DYM. (2006) New insights into the complex gene-environment interactions evolving into atopic dermatitis. *J Allergy Clin Immunol* **118**: 37–39.

Flohr C, Johansson SGO, Wahlgren C-F. (2004) How atopic is atopic dermatitis? *J Allergy Clin Immunol* **114**: 150–158.

Dekio I, Sakamoto M, Hayashi H, *et al.* (2007) Characterization of skin microbiota in patients with atopic dermatitis and in normal subjects using 16S rRNA gene-based comprehensive analysis. *J Med Microbiol* **56**: 1675–1683

Allam JP and Novak N. (2006) The pathophysiology of atopic eczema. *Clin Exp Dermatol* **31**: 89–93.

Cai SC, Chen H, Koh WP. (2012) Filaggrin mutations are associated with recurrent skin infection in Singaporean Chinese patients with atopic dermatitis. *Br J Dermatol* **166**: 200–203.

Werfel T, Ballmer-Weber B, Eigenmann PA, *et al.* (2007) Worm M. Eczematous reactions to food in atopic eczema: position paper of the EAACI and GA2LEN. *Allergy* **62**: 723–728.

7. Diagnosis–Tests

Diagnostic features of atopic dermatitis. Acta Dermatol Venereol (Stockh) 1980, 92, 44–47.

Wüthrich B. Unproven techniques in allergy diagnosis. J Invest Allergol Clin Immunol 2005, 15, 86–90.

Libeer J-C, Van Hoeyveld E, Kochuyt A-M, Weykamp C, Bossuyt X. In vitro determination of allergen-specific serum IgE. Comparative analysis of three methods. Clin Chem Lab Med 2007, 45, 413–415.

Glovsky MM. Measuring allergen specific IgE: where have we been and where are we going now? Methods Mol Biol 2007, 378, 205–219.

8. Prevention of Eczema

Bertelsen RJ, Brantsæter AL, Magnus MC, Haugen M, Myhre R, Jacobsson B, Longnecker MP, Meltzer HM, London SJ. Probiotic milk consumption in pregnancy and infancy and subsequent childhood allergic diseases. *J Allergy Clin Immunol.* 2013 Sep 10. pii: S0091–6749 (13)01157–3

Osborn DA, Sinn J. Formulas containing hydrolysed protein for prevention of allergy and food intolerance in infants. *Cochrane Database Syst Rev.* 2006 Oct 18;(4):CD003664.

Isolauri E, Salminen S; Nutrition, Allergy, Mucosal Immunology, and Intestinal Microbiota (NAMI) Research Group Report. Probiotics: use in allergic disorders: a Nutrition, Allergy, Mucosal Immunology, and Intestinal Microbiota (NAMI) Research Group Report. *J Clin Gastroenterol* 2008, 42 Suppl 2, S91–6.

Kalliomäki M, Salminen S, Arvilommi H, Kero P, Koskinen P, Isolauri E. Probiotics in primary prevention of atopic disease: A randomized placebo-controlled trial. *Lancet* 2001, 357, 1076–1079.

Taylor AT, Dunstan JA, Prescott SL. Probiotic supplementation for the first 6 months of life fails to reduce the risk of atopic dermatitis and increases the risk of allergen sensitization in high-risk children: a randomized controlled trial. *J Allergy Clin Immunol* 2007, 119, 184–191.

Moro S, Arslanoglu S, Stahl B, *et al.* (2006) A mixture of prebiotic oligosaccharides reduces the incidence of atopic dermatitis during the first six months of age. *Arch Dis Childh* 91: 814–819.

9. Treatment of Eczema

Akdis CA, Adkis M, Bieber T *et al.* (2006) European Academy of Allergology; Clinical Immunology / American Academy of Allergy, Asthma and immunology/ PRACTALL Consensus Report. *Allergy* 61: 969–987.

Sang-Il Lee, Jihyun Kim, Youngshin Han and Kangmo Ahn. (2011) A proposal: Atopic Dermatitis Organizer (ADO) guideline for children. *Asia Pac Allergy* 1: 53–63.

Belloni B, Andres C, Ollert M, *et al.* (2008) Novel immunological approaches in the treatment of atopic eczema. *Curr Opin Allergy Clin Immunol* 8: 423–427.

10. Prognosis and Long-Term Evolution

von Kobyletzki LB, Bornehag CG, Breeze E, *et al.* (2013) Factors Associated with Remission of Eczema in Children: a Population-based Follow-up Study. *Acta Derm Venereol* Sep 16. doi: 10.2340/00015555–1681.

Carlsten C, *et al.* (2013) Atopic dermatitis in a high-risk cohort: natural history, associated allergic outcomes, and risk factors. *Ann Allergy Asthma Immunol* **110**: 24–28.

van der Hulst AE, Klip H, Brand PLP. (2007) Risk of developing asthma in young children with atopic eczema: A systematic review. *J Allergy Clin Immunol* **120**: 565–569.

11. Future Research

Van Bever HP, Lee BW, Shek L. (2012) Viewpoint: the future of research in pediatric allergy: what should the focus be? *Pediatr Allergy Immunol* **23**: 5–10.

Index